Population Economics

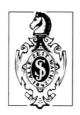

Jacques J. Siegers · Jenny de Jong-Gierveld
Evert van Imhoff (Eds.)

Female Labour Market Behaviour and Fertility

A Rational-Choice Approach

Proceedings of a Workshop Organized by the
Netherlands Interdisciplinary Demographic Institute (NIDI)
in Collaboration with the Economic Institute /
Centre for Interdisciplinary Research on Labour Market
and Distribution Issues (CIAV) of Utrecht University
Held in The Hague, The Netherlands, April 20-22, 1989

With 13 Figures

Springer-Verlag Berlin Heidelberg New York London
Paris Tokyo Hong Kong Barcelona Budapest

Prof. Dr. Jacques J. Siegers
Economic Institute / Centre for Interdisciplinary Research
on Labour Market and Distribution Issues (CIAV)
Utrecht University
Domplein 24
3512 JE Utrecht, The Netherlands

Prof. Dr. Jenny de Jong-Gierveld
Dr. Evert van Imhoff
Netherlands Interdisciplinary
Demographic Institute (NIDI)
P.O. Box 11650
2502 AR The Hague, The Netherlands

ISBN 3-540-53896-8 Springer-Verlag Berlin Heidelberg New York Tokyo
ISBN 0-387-53896-8 Springer-Verlag New York Heidelberg Berlin Tokyo

© Springer-Verlag Berlin · Heidelberg 1991
Printed in Germany

Printing: Weihert-Druck GmbH, Darmstadt
Bookbinding: J. Schäffer GmbH u. Co. KG, Grünstadt
2142/7130-543210

PREFACE

Since 1987, the investigation of the relationship between female labour market behaviour and fertility, which forms part of the research programme of the Economic Institute / Centre for Interdisciplinary Research on Labour Market and Distribution Issues (CIAV) of Utrecht University, also became a part of the research programme of the Netherlands Interdisciplinary Demographic Institute (NIDI). Since then, I have been entrusted with research on this topic. In this context, I acted on a suggestion made by Frans Willekens to organize an international workshop, with the help of other members of the NIDI staff and with the administrative and organizational support of the NIDI.

This resulted in the workshop "Female Labour Market Behaviour and Fertility: Preferences, Restrictions, Behaviour," held at the Netherlands Interdisciplinary Demographic Institute in The Hague, April 20-22, 1989, under the auspices of the European Association for Population Studies (EAPS). In this workshop, demographers, econometricians, economists, psychologists and socio-logists discussed the paths to a truly interdisciplinary approach to the relationship between female labour market behaviour and fertility. Such an interdisciplinary approach requires a common theoretical framework. The rational-choice framework was considered to be best suited to this purpose. As a consequence, the workshop was not only structured by *what* was studied, but also by *how* it was studied.

This volume consists of the papers presented at the above-mentioned workshop, as revised by the authors in collaboration with the editors. Financial support for the workshop and the publication of this book by the Netherlands Ministry of Social Affairs and Employment, by the Netherlands Ministry of Education and Sciences, and by the Royal Netherlands Academy of Sciences (KNAW) is gratefully acknowledged, as well as the co-operative efforts of the NIDI-staff (in particular ms. Mariette van Woensel) and of my colleague-editors.

August 1990   Jacques J. Siegers

CONTENTS

EDITORS' INTRODUCTION

Jacques J. Siegers, Jenny de Jong-Gierveld and Evert van Imhoff
Nederlands Interdisciplinair Demografisch Instituut
P.O. Box 11650
2502 AR THE HAGUE
The Netherlands

This volume contains the papers presented at the conference "Female Labour Market Behaviour and Fertility: Preferences, Restrictions, Behaviour," held in April 1989 at the Netherlands Interdisciplinary Demographic Institute in The Hague. It is often suggested that the increased labour force participation of women in the West has played an important role in reducing fertility and that fertility may continue to decrease if the growth in female labour force participation persists. However, the economic and socio-demographic literature indicates that this causality is not as evident as many people believe. This means that we cannot be sure that measures aimed at creating better opportunities for women to combine parenthood and paid labour will actually influence fertility and if they do, what the influence will be. In order to be able to answer questions such as those regarding the effects of policy measures, further theoretical and empirical interdisciplinary research will have to be carried out into the relationship between female labour force participation and fertility. The workshop aimed to contribute to this research.

The term "interdisciplinary" used above refers to the integration of various disciplinary approaches within one theoretical framework, as opposed to a multidisciplinary approach in which the problem is studied in various separate disciplines. The theoretical framework used in the workshop is a *rational-choice framework*. It is assumed that human behaviour can be explained with the aid of a "preferences - restrictions - behaviour" scheme. Human beings are assumed to be led by preferences, and to strive towards maximum realization of their preferences. Due to restrictions, which force people to make choices, preferences can never fully be realized. Behaviour is the outcome of this process.

It was the purpose of the workshop to use the rational-choice framework as an engine to integrate the contributions of the participants who represented the fields of demography, econometrics, economics, psychology and sociology. In line with this purpose, the participants were asked to approach the subject from their own discipline in such a way that the different elements of the "preferences - restrictions - behaviour" scheme were filled. The aim was to contribute to the construction of a sound foundation for empirical analyses with the aid of surveys, to the further development of theories and empirical analytical methods, and to the evaluation of policy measures.

In line with the structure of the workshop, this volume consists of five parts: I) Theoretical Points of Departure; II) Preferences; III) Restrictions; IV) Confrontation of Preferences and Restrictions: The Construction of Theoretical Models; V) Towards a Better Understanding of the Interrelationship between Female Labour Market Behaviour and Fertility.

Part I, *Theoretical Points of Departure*, consists of two papers that provide a basic and coherent introduction to the study of female labour market behaviour and fertility with the use of the rational-choice framework: *Understanding the Interdependence between Parallel Careers* by Frans Willekens, and *Social Approval, Fertility and Female Labour Market Behaviour* by Siegwart Lindenberg.

Understanding the Interdependence between Parallel Careers starts with a concise review of recent research on the relationship between female employment and fertility. Frans Willekens establishes that the available findings are inconsistent. He suggests a process approach to integrate the various research findings within a common framework. According to this approach, observed patterns of fertility and employment are outcomes of parallel career processes, which continuously interact with each other and with their common environment. In these career processes, the interaction concerns available resources: an individual has a limited amount of time and energy to allocate to family and work. Moreover, both careers are in their critical stages at about the same point in time. If the two careers are to be combined, the incompatibility needs to be resolved, either by appropriate timing of the life events (e.g. births, labour market entries and exits) or through the provision of additional resources by others (by members of the support network or by the formal sector).

Willekens not only stresses the process character of the relationship between female labour market behaviour and fertility, but also indicates that the behavioural patterns under discussion can only be understood by identifying and describing the mental processes that govern these patterns. The author expects the impact of personality development on demographic behaviour to become stronger.

In his paper *Social Approval, Fertility and Female Labour Market Behaviour*, Siegwart Lindenberg introduces a number of traditional sociological insights (especially those concerning the importance of social approval) into the economic model-building approach to the relationship between work and family. The author emphasizes the importance of a constraint-driven heuristic, with general human goals (namely physical well-being and social approval) and social production functions as means for reaching these goals. As a basis for the formulation of the relevant social production functions, he starts with what may be called the fundamental exchange, resting on two assumptions: a) a "home" is of fundamental importance for the production of physical well-being; and b) with the exception of some complementary activities, there are gains from specialization in making a home and in providing the means for making a home, leading to a division of labour between the specialists. The fundamental exchange is the exchange between the specialists: "making a home" in exchange for "providing the means for making a home" and vice versa. Given the well-known division of labour between the sexes, the social production function for physical well-being for men contains "providing the means for making a home" and "making use of the home," and for women it contains "making use of the means provided for making a home", "making a home" and "making use of the home." Next, Lindenberg establishes several elements of the social production function for social approval, and sketches the workings of different forms of social approval with regard to family and labour market. These results enable one to investigate the considerable changes in female labour market behaviour and fertility, and to detect the privatization of consumption and the resulting erosion of social norms as one of the determinants of these changes.

Part II, *Preferences*, involves four papers: *De Gustibus Confusi Sumus ?* by Thomas Burch, *Shortcuts as Pitfalls ? Ways of Measuring Childbearing Preferences and Intentions* by Freddy Deven and Sabien Bauwens, *Motivation for Reproductive Behaviour and the Professional Motivation of Women* by Erika Spieß, Friedemann Nerdinger and Lutz von Rosenstiel, and *A Purposeful Behaviour Theory of Work and Family Size Decisions* by Richard Bagozzi and Frances Van Loo.

The central thesis of Thomas Burch's paper *De Gustibus Confusi Sumus ?* is that the concept of preferences continues to be used indiscriminately to refer to a number of conceptually distinct subjective states of respondents which also prove to be empirically distinct. In other words, the element "preferences" from the "preferences - restrictions - behaviour" scheme needs a thorough process of conceptualization and operationalization, as well as a valid and reliable measurement instrument to be used in survey research. The arguments are illustrated with examples taken from the 1984 Canadian Fertility Survey.

Surveys cost time and money. Freddy Deven and Sabien Bauwens, in their paper *Shortcuts as Pitfalls ? Ways of Measuring Childbearing Preferences and Intentions*, investigate whether piecemeal measurement of the increasingly sophisticated models to study reproductive behaviour produces incomplete and/or biased knowledge, using data from Flanders Surveys on Family Development. They stress the importance of having a specific theoretical framework as the basis for data collection.

Erika Spieß, Friedemann Nerdinger and Lutz von Rosenstiel present, in their paper *Motivation for Reproductive Behaviour and the Professional Motivation of Women*, a couple-interaction-model of reproductive behaviour. The starting point of this model is the individual value structure of the husband and wife. Using data from a sample of young married German women, the importance of values for reproductive behaviour is demonstrated.

According to Richard Bagozzi and Frances Van Loo, early research efforts attempting to identify the psychological determinants of fertility and efforts to explain career orientation as a function of psychological variables were not successful, due to a lack of a well-developed theory and of adequate measurement techniques. Although, beginning in the 1970s and continuing into the 1980s, the application of the expectancy-value model, which was based on firmer theoretical grounds than earlier approaches and which was accompanied by relatively more accurate measurement techniques, produced results that were much improved, there are still many shortcomings. In their paper *A Purposeful Behaviour Theory of Work and Family Size Decisions*, Bagozzi and Van Loo develop a theory that builds upon the expectancy-value model, yet goes well beyond it in form and substance. One of the premises of their theory is that the fullest explanation of work and family size decisions rests on the specification of the elementary psychological processes going on withing the bodies and minds of men and women, as well as of the social-psychological processes transpiring between them as they socially construct their life experiences. Many theories in the social sciences have ignored these processes by focussing only upon the associations between inputs (e.g. income, education) and outputs (e.g. employment, family size). In contrast, Bagozzi and Van Loo try to specify the intervening mechanisms.

Part III, *Restrictions*, contains two papers: *A Biographic/Demographic Analysis of the Relationship between Fertility and Occupational Activity of Women and Married Couples* by Herwig Birg, and *Labour Market Restrictions and the Role of Preferences in Family Economics* by Klaus Zimmermann and John De New.

In his paper *A Biographic/Demographic Analysis of the Relationship between Fertility and Occupational Activity of Women and Married Couples*, Herwig Birg applies the analytical tools of the biographic theory of fertility to the analysis of interdependencies between life course events that are usually treated separately by economists on the one hand and sociologists on the other hand. Biographies are regarded as the outcome of dynamic decision processes. Present choices affect the range of future opportunities. However, in the dynamic processes preferences and restrictions may change their parts. As is illustrated in the paper, the biographic approach can be interpreted as a method of applying the "preferences - restrictions - behaviour" scheme to the problem of biographic sequences.

Klaus Zimmermann and John De New present in their paper *Labour Market Restrictions and the Role of Preferences in Family Economics* a simple economic model in which labour supply and fertility are jointly determined. They show that labour market conditions are decisive in determining fertility. Using starting values that are rationed with respect to labour, preferences even prove to play no role in determining fertility whatsoever. Furthermore, the authors conjecture that fertility decline is a more likely event in the process of economic growth if labour supply is rationed.

Part IV, *Confrontation of Preferences and Restrictions: The Construction of Theoretical Models*, comprises four papers: *Economic Models of Women's Employment and Fertility* by John Ermisch, the twin papers by Alice Nakamura and Masao Nakamura on *Models of Female Labour Market Supply, with Special Reference to the Effects of Children* and *Children and Female Labour Market Supply: A Survey of Econometric Approaches*, and the paper *How Economics, Psychology and Sociology Might Produce a Unified Theory of Fertility and Labour Force Participation* by Boone Turchi.

The paper *Economic Models of Women's Employment and Fertility* by John Ermisch is a review of economic studies of women's labour supply and fertility. The author concludes that there have been relatively few contributions of new models to guide the empirical analysis since the classic study of Willis (1974); the primary contribution of recent studies is in the model's econometric estimation. He also concludes that both static and dynamic economic models are easily accomodated to comply with the "preferences - restrictions - behaviour" scheme of the present volume.

In their paper *Models of Female Labour Market Supply, with Special Reference to the Effects of Children*, Alice and Masao Nakamura point to the fact that children have at least two kinds of effects on female labour supply. First, there are the direct effects, i.e. the effects on female labour supply of the time, expenditure and effort needed to bear and raise children. Second, there are the indirect effects, i.e. the effects of human capital accumulation transmitted via the wage offers women receive. The indirect effects of children on female labour supply are, of course, determined by the extent to which female labour supply is responsive to current period or intertemporal offered wage rates. The authors note that especially in the earlier economic literature on female labour supply, the child-related effects are treated as nuisance factors that have to be controlled in order to obtain efficient and consistent estimates of the income and substitution effects, while more recently there has been increased interest in child status effects in their own right.

In their companion paper *Children and Female Labour Market Supply: A Survey of Econometric Approaches*, Alice and Masao Nakamura discuss a number of basic econometric choices concerning the limited nature of the dependent variables in models of female labour supply, sample selection bias, and bias problems associated with specific explanatory variables. They find that direct child-related effects are quantitatively more important on female labour market participation than they are on the hours of work for women with paid jobs. Both economic theory and available empirical results suggest that women's child bearing and rearing roles are responsible, to some degree, for the observed wage disadvantage of working women versus working men. However, the empirical evidence on the wage response of labour supply suggests that the indirect effects of children on the hours of work of working women (as opposed to the probability of work) are probably modest. They note that little is known yet about the importance of indirect child-related effects on labour market participation, largely because information on wage offers is usually available only for those women who work.

Boone Turchi argues in his paper *How Economics, Psychology and Sociology Might Produce a Unified Theory of Fertility and Labour Force Participation* that the microeconomic model as usually employed can serve a potentially valuable role as an integrating framework for the interdisciplinary study of fertility and labour force participation behaviour, by integrating economic as well as psychological and sociological variables to produce a comprehensive model. The model presented by Turchi in his paper reflects the author's conviction that the fertility-labour force participation relationship must be treated as short run behaviour conditioned by long run plans.

In part V, the "Closing Section", in his paper *Towards a Better Understanding of the Interrelationship between Female Labour Market Behaviour and Fertility*, Jacques Siegers presents concise evaluations of the economic approaches to labour supply and fertility, respectively. He also sketches how within the rational-choice framework, the "preferences - restrictions - behaviour" scheme can be used as a basis for an interdisciplinary analysis of the relationship between female labour market behaviour and fertility.

The results of the workshop "Female Labour Market Behaviour and Fertility: Preferences, Restrictions, Behaviour", as presented in this volume, are being implemented in a survey project which is currently conducted by the Economic Institute / Centre for Interdisciplinary Research on Labour Market and Distribution Issues (CIAV) of Utrecht University, and the Netherlands Inter-disciplinary Demographic Institute (NIDI). The project is funded by the Netherlands Organization for Scientific Research (NWO). Our experience is that the results of the workshop are of great significance to the afore-mentioned project. We hope and trust that the same holds for survey projects in other countries and that the present volume may lead to a better understanding of the relationship between female labour market behaviour and fertility.

Part I
Theoretical Points of Departure

UNDERSTANDING THE INTERDEPENDENCE BETWEEN PARALLEL CAREERS

Frans J. Willekens
Nederlands Interdisciplinair Demografisch Instituut
P.O. Box 11650
2502 AR   THE HAGUE
The Netherlands

2.1. Introduction

"Scientific inquiry is concerned not only with discovering quantitative relations between variables, but also with interpreting these relations in terms of underlying causal mechanisms that produced them. Without a knowledge of these mechanisms, we cannot predict how variables will co-vary when the structure of the system under study is altered, either experimentally or by changes in the world around us." (Simon, 1979, p. 79). Increasingly, demographers emphasize the need to identify the underlying or intervening mechanisms linking demographic variables and suggest ways to accomplish the difficult task (Burch, 1980, p. 2; Caldwell and Hill, 1988, p. 1; Birg, 1988). The search for causal mechanisms is part of an attempt to develop a substantive theory of demographic behaviour. This paper is written in the same spirit. The aim is to explore the nature of the interdependencies between parallel careers. The fertility and labour force participation careers of women serve as an example. For no other set of two careers, the interdependence is as pronounced as for the fertility and employment careers. The basis for the interdependence is generally conflict or incompatibility, because "the timing of critical career-building phases does not accommodate women's biological life cycle" (Regan and Roland, 1985, p. 986).

Recent research findings on the interdependence between fertility and labour force participation are reviewed in section 2. The findings are inconsistent. In order to integrate the various research findings in a common framework we suggest a process approach. Employment and fertility are parallel processes, which interact with each other. The process perspective raises some new issues of causality. They are discussed in section 3. Sections 4, 5 and 6 present the main theory proposed in this paper to understand the interdependence between parallel careers. A main thesis is that relations between variables pertaining to fertility and employment are mediated by personality traits, in particular the career orientations. The theory is applied to the study of the fertility-employment interaction in section 7. Section 8 concludes the paper.

2.2. Fertility and employment: a few research findings

Many studies indicate the existence of effects of family responsibilities on women's paid work and vice versa.[1] The Population Conference organized by the United Nations in Sofia (1983) reached the conclusion that "A number of delegates referred to the increasing participation of women in the labor force as one of the major factors in the decline of fertility" (United Nations, 1983, p. 6). Waite *et al.* (1984), summarizing previous research on the relationship between fertility and employment, arrive at the opposite conclusion: "Fertility influences work but work has no measurable impact on fertility." Klijzing *et al.* (1988) arrive at the same conclusion after applying three different methodologies to a single set of data from a retrospective survey (ORIN), which lead them to conclude that the decision to have a(nother) child is taken independently from labour force participation decisions.

Other authors would qualify these statements. Siegers (1985, p. 318) finds that the negative effect of the presence of children on labour force participation of married women is larger if the children are younger. The effect is, however, reduced if there are older children in the family. Personal characteristics such as level of education may affect the relationship (see e.g. Bernhardt, 1986). Nakamura and Nakamura (1984a) suggest that the effect of fertility on labour force participation is an artefact of cross-sectional studies. Using longitudinal data, they show that the impact on current work behaviour of the presence of children and of birth expectations is almost entirely reflected in a woman's work behaviour in previous years. Calhoun and Espenshade (1988, p. 29) and Veron (1988, p. 108) also find that cross-sectional studies overestimate the effect of fertility on labour force participation. Using French census data for the period 1962-1982, Veron finds that the participation rate of women increased irrespective of the number of

---

[1] Extensive reviews of research are: Spitze (1988) for US studies; Siegers (1985) and Mol *et al.* (1988. pp. 3-7) for Dutch studies; Standing (1978, pp. 192 ff.) for studies in developing countries.

children present. Women with no or few children are involved more in paid labour, but so are women with large families.

Unobservable attributes, mainly psychological in nature, such as "desire for motherhood" and other personality traits are also introduced to explain observed interaction. Ermisch (this volume, chapter 10) relies on this variable to explain that, among married childless women, those not in full-time jobs are much more likely to conceive. Additional examples are given in Section 7.

A few authors explicitly introduce the person's ability to think prospectively. Greene and Quester (1982) and Johnson and Skinner (1985), for instance, find that wives' labour supply is affected positively by the perceived risk of marital dissolution (see also Davis, 1984). This result of micro-level analysis is consistent with Fuchs' finding that the rise in labour force participation by married women with small children at home preceded by several years the rise in the divorce rate (Fuchs, 1983, p. 149). In an extensive review of research on the effects of women's employment on families, Spitze concludes that the analysis of behaviour suggests that the causal ordering is from fertility to employment, but that employment plans or intentions affect expected fertility more than the reverse (Spitze, 1988, p. 606).

Bulatao and Fawcett (1981, p. 437) find empirical support for their hypothesis that women with higher occupational aspirations are more likely to postpone early childbearing in order to get ahead in their occupational careers. They also find support for the hypothesis that early experience affects subsequent behaviour: women who have their first child at a younger age generally have more children and at shorter intervals. Teachman and Heckert (1985) find, however, that the effect of first-birth timing on subsequent childspacing has declined in more recent cohorts, showing that the "early-pregnancy treadmill" is losing its significance. The effect of early experience on subsequent behaviour also applies to the work career: women who worked before having children are more likely to work again at any time later in their lives than women who did not acquire work experience before having children (Mott, 1972; Mott and Shapiro, 1983).

In her study "The changing role of women in the British labour market and the family", Joshi (1988) summarizes the reasons why a woman is more likely to engage in paid work: rising levels of education, changes in attitudes, rising risk of divorce, improved health of women and children and improved technology of housework.

In order to explore the causal mechanism that underlies the observed interdependence between motherhood and employment, we view labour force participation and childbearing as *two parallel career processes*, which interact with each other and with their common environment. It is believed that both career activities are organized by a common dynamic mechanism which will be referred to as the *coordinating process*. The coordinating process is the process of human development and is related to Erikson's (1980) notion that life is a quest for identity and to Maslow's (1954, 1973) notion of self-actualization and self-determination (autonomy). But first a few statements on causality are in order. Conventional criteria for causality may not be valid in case processes are studied.

2.3. A note on causality

Two important criteria for causality do not necessarily apply in case of interacting processes. They are the conditions of *temporal ordering* and *contiguity*. Causes are required to occur prior to their effects. This requirement seemingly conflicts with the fact that human beings can think prospectively. They can form expectations of future events or conditions, anticipate consequences of actions and plan for the future. Simon (1979, p. 73) argues that this is not a case of the future influencing the present, because the expectations and anticipations are not actually determined by future events or conditions but by current knowledge that is predictive of the events or conditions. In other words, present behaviour is determined by predictions of the future, rather than by the future itself. The temporal order in which behaviour occurs is therefore often not a good indicator of causal priority. The causal priority is established in the mind in a way that is not reflected in the temporal sequence of behaviour (Marini and Singer, 1988, p. 377). For instance, consider the relationship between labour force participation and marital status. Among married women who enter or reenter the labour force prior to divorce, there are some who will enter the labour force and then decide to divorce and others who will decide to divorce and then look for a job in anticipation of the impending divorce. For the former group, labour force entry is causally prior to divorce; for the latter group, the divorce is causally prior to labour force entry. Since the anticipation of divorce may affect labour force behaviour prior to divorce, the temporal ordering of the events does not reflect the causal priority. Martini and Singer argue that this problem is not necessarily solved by considering the temporal sequence of the formation of the behavioural intentions. When there is a perceived incompatibility between future activities, a single decision may jointly produce a related set of behavioural intentions. Causal priority can only be identified by asking people about the causal processes at work (Marini and Singer, 1988, p. 378). This, however, requires in-depth interviewing; records of the sequence and timing of overt behaviour are not sufficient.

The second requirement is that cause and effect be contiguous. In the tradition of the philosopher Hume, contiguity in space and time is a criterion of causation since contiguity makes structural continuity possible. The condition of contiguity of cause and effect is frequently not met in dynamic processes for two reasons. First, an "incubation period" may be required for the effect to become manifest. In addition, the effect may be spread out over time. Second, the dependence between two processes may be governed by a third, intervening process upon which the processes are jointly dependent. The intervening process serves the function of a causal process in Salmon's theory of scientific inference (Salmon, 1984; see also Marini and Singer, 1988, pp. 361 ff.). A causal process is capable of transmitting structure and modifications in structure and is therefore "capable of propagating a causal influence from one space-time locate to another" (Salmon, 1984, p. 155). The causal process connects two processes and explains their relationship. The contiguity requirement is untenable in life course analysis, because it does not allow a causal link between childhood experience and adult behaviour. The link does exist although it is not a direct one; the effect of early experience can be substantially modified by later experiences. Runyan's formulation fits nicely in the context of this paper: "The effects of early experiences are mediated through a chain of behavior-determining, person-determining and situation-determining processes throughout the life course." (Runyan, 1984, p. 212).

2.4. Human development: the temporal dimension

The British Medical Dictionary defines development as "The series of changes by which the individual embryo becomes a mature organism" (Sinclair, 1985, p. 1). Development implies evolution: new functions are acquired and old ones are lost. In Maslow's view, the evolution is towards self-actualization and self-realization. Maslow (1954, 1973) segregates and orders different sets of human needs according to the immediacy with which their satisfaction is required (figure 1).

Basic physiological needs are the most pressing and fundamental ones, and their satisfaction is seen as prerequisite to seeking the satisfaction of the safety needs on the next higher level. Satisfaction of the safety needs is, in turn, prerequisite to seeking the satisfaction of self-esteem needs and self-actualization. The needs provide the motives for behaviour. In general, persons will try to achieve higher-order needs when conditions permit. Two needs are of particular relevance in the study of the interdependence between work and family careers. They are "protection from immediate or future threat to economic well-being" (safety need) and "self-actualization." Work for financial reasons is associated with the first need, while work for autonomy

Figure 1. Maslow's hierarchy of human needs

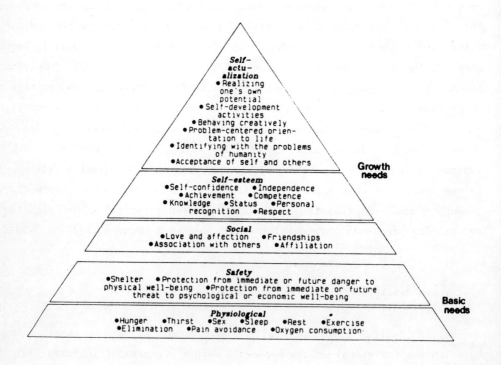

Source: Ickes, 1985, p. 6.

relates to the second aspiration, which is the highest in the hierarchy. The distinction between the two needs is the distinction between necessity and choice.

Developmental goals are dynamic. They change with the changing person and are affected by the environment. The context in which a person lives helps to shape the goals and facilitates or constrains their achievement (Lerner and Kauffman, 1985). In a choice framework, the context determines the extent to which a person is free to establish priorities and to allocate time and energy accordingly. In other words, it defines the options among which a person may choose (choice set). Biological, normative, economic, physical and situational factors affect the ability to achieve the goals or satisfy the needs. The context is composed of multiple levels changing interdependently across time (i.e. historically). Two levels of context are distinguished. The micro-context consists of the living and work environment and the people with whom personal relationships are maintained. The macro-context is the social, cultural and economic system, which determines the historical context in which a person lives. The micro-context can be influenced by the person, but the macro-context cannot.

To describe and interpret human behaviour, behavioural and social scientists increasingly rely on a developmental perspective. What distinguishes development studies from other studies of behaviour is that they are concerned with behavioural *sequences* and with the *processes* that underlie overt behaviour. A particular stimulus may trigger a behavioural pattern consisting of several changes (events or actions). A single decision may involve several actions. The developmental perspective emphasizes that changes or actions are related and contribute to and are affected by development.

Development is a continuous, however not monotonous, process. The life events that characterize human development are not uniformly distributed over the lifespan, but are concentrated in relatively short periods and constitute an orderly sequence. Each stage of development is characterized by a particular potential for development or developmental readiness, as referred to by Erikson (1980). Infancy, adolescence, young adult, adulthood, and mature age are examples of stages that are frequently distinguished in the psychological literature. Individuals go through the stages in infinitely varied ways, but the stages themselves are universal. The stages are separated by relatively short periods of transition. The chain of stable periods and transition periods pertaining to a given domain of life is referred to as a *career*. Careers that are distinguished relate to profession, employment, fertility, education, health, place of residence, etc. A career can be associated with each attribute of a person that changes over the lifetime (Willekens, 1988). Careers may be characterized by the type of transitions or events that occur and by the pattern of occurrences (sequence and timing).

Transitions are generally preceded by transitional periods. These boundary zones between stable periods serve important functions in human development. During these periods, the question "Who am I ?", which is generally associated with the quest for identity, is augmented by the question "Where am I ?." Life commitments and activities are questioned and reappraised, new career options are explored, different directions are experimented with and, finally, choices are made. The very nature of the transitional period results in unstable commitments and unstable choices (Van Geert, 1986, p. 31). A transitional period is required to summarize, evaluate and terminate the past and to start the future (Levinson *et al.*, 1978, p. 50; Levinson and Gooden, 1985, p. 6; see also Plath, 1983, p. 48). The onset of the period is characterized by a dis-satisfaction or conflict. The period is completed when career choices are made and a commitment to adhere to the choices is reached. During the subsequent stable period, the changes are consolidated and a new life structure is built.

Needs pertaining to the various life domains are not given and fixed, but they develop as a result of continuous interaction between the person and the context, in particular the society in which a person lives. From the values and needs, a person derives career orientations or attitudes. A career is a route to goal-achievement. It is, therefore, not only a sequence of events and stages, but it is a goal-directed or purposive sequence. The career *orientation* represents the attitudinal dimension or the predisposition to engage in a career. It may be viewed as being determined by two factors: the belief that engaging in a career brings about certain consequences (expectancy) and the contribution of the consequences to the fulfillment of the needs (value or anticipated life satisfaction). This view is consistent with the value-expectancy theory and provides a possibility to add a time dimension to this theory. The orientation or attitude provides the motives to become involved in a career. This involvement is denoted by career *commitment*. Commitment requires a person to allocate adequate time and energy. The higher the commitment to a career, the more time and energy is allocated. If external constraints permit, commitment results in career *attachment*, which refers to the person's behaviour over time. This distinction between career orientation, commitment and attachment is not universally accepted. The concepts are usually loosely defined in the literature and that hinders the progress in life course theory. There have been attempts to clarify the concepts, but the outcome is not fully satisfactory (Hiller and Dyehouse, 1987).

2.5. Human development: parallel processes

Life consists of many domains. The activities pertaining to the various domains are overlapping. The career processes associated with the domains are active simultaneously and they interact with each other and with their common environment. The nature and the extent of the interdependence are very difficult to identify in the real world. Processes may depend on each other directly or indirectly through a third process. The impact of one process on another may become manifest after a long time only. Ideally, the study of the dependence structure involves first the isolation of each process from the influences of concurrent processes, as is done in a laboratory context and the study of the dynamics of the process "in a pure state", i.e. undisturbed by the presence of other processes. Once the intrinsic properties of each process are revealed, any set of processes may be combined to find out how they interact. These experiments are not feasible yet, so we are left with the study of interacting processes "in situ" and cannot do much more than hypothesize about the mechanisms by which career processes interact. We assume that the careers pertain to the same person.

Three types of dependencies between career processes are distinguished: *event dependence*, *status dependence* and *resource dependence*.

Event dependence
Career A is said to be event-dependent on career B if the occurrence of an event in career A, implying an advancement or progression, is influenced by the occurrence of an event in career B. The event in B may enhance or inhibit the occurrence of an event in A. It may also make the occurrence of an event possible. For instance, most professions require a diploma. The onset of the professional career is therefore contingent upon the completion of formal education. Some events involve two processes. Marriage, for instance, involves the marital career of two persons. An extreme case of event-dependence occurs when a career is truncated by an event in another career. Death for instance,

which is the event in the survival process, interrupts all existing careers. The advancement of any career is contingent upon the person being alive (the survival process being intact).

Status dependence

Career A is status-dependent on career B if the occurrence of an event in career A depends on the position (stage) occupied in career B. For instance, the probability of having a child in a given year depends on the marital status.

Resource dependence

Careers A and B are resource-dependent if they share the same resource. If the two careers together use less resources than when they operate separately, the dependence is referred to as symbiosis: the careers are complementary. If, on the other hand, they compete for the same limited resources, the careers are conflicting or incompatible. For instance, work and family careers are conflicting careers, since both require time and energy (resources) for their advancement.

The assumption that the careers pertain to the same person is important. Career processes in different persons may interact too, and the type of dependence may be one of the three listed. But the interaction is mediated by the personal relationship, in particular by the information channels that are established as part of the relationship. The flow of information (communication) becomes a critical component of the dependence structure.

The dependence structure is assumed to be organized hierarchically. For simplicity, we assume a single coordinating process which mediates the onset and progression of all processes. Other authors consider several coordinating processes.

The conceptual framework presented in this paper views overt behaviour as an outcome of a complex set of interconnected mental processes. The processes are organized hierarchically. High in the hierarchy are processes that relate to domains with the greatest significance for the self and the life course. These processes, which are referred to as *dominant processes*, are directly connected to the coordinating process. The other, *secondary processes* are linked indirectly to the coordinating process.

The hierarchical organization of processes has important consequences for the scheduling of events across the career processes. If a career process is subordinate to another career process, its events are scheduled to meet the requirements of the dominant career. For instance, if the family career is subordinate to the work career, family planning must make allowance for the work schedule.

The transitional period serves to build a new hierarchy of career processes by making choices about aspects of the greatest personal significance. The aspects pertain to domains - generally one or two, rarely as many as three - that occupy a central place in the life structure. Most often, marriage, family and occupation are the central domains. They receive the largest share of ones's time and energy, and they strongly influence the character of the other domains. Once choices about the most significant domains are made, the conflicts in other careers sharing the same resources may more easily be resolved. Sometimes events occur "off-time", before the period of developmental readiness is reached, and affect all career processes. If such an occurrence is in a career that demands resources, the consequence may be a lifetime of stress. Premature pregnancy serves as an illustration. It "tends to disrupt and accelerate the life cycle of the adolescent by pre-empting educational, vocational and social experiences of persons at an early stage in their life" (Van den Akker, 1988, p. 327). The lifetime consequences are documented by Van den Akker.

2.6. The coordinating process

Several authors have suggested some sort of coordinating process that controls the various processes that characterize ageing and the life course and ensures an orderly sequence of events. Although the process has a considerable autonomy, it is affected by stimuli from other processes and the environment. Biologists believe that the coordination is taken care of by a sensor or regulator, which is biological in nature, and an ageing clock, which is genetic. The environment affects the timing of the ageing clock through an ageing centre, where the sensory inputs of temperature, nutrition, hormone information, etc. are assessed and the appropriate signal is transmitted to the clock (Everitt, 1982; Moore-Ede *et al.*, 1982). Sociologists believe that the main regulator of the timing of life events consists of a normative prescription. The "proper" timing of life events and the duration of stages between events are viewed as an important instrument of social control and a stabilizing factor in social structure (Elchardus, 1984; Roth, 1963, 1983). The existence of a "proper" order of events and of socially expected durations induces Zerubavel to suggest that "we carry in our minds a sort of 'temporal map', which consists of all our expectations regarding the sequential order, duration, temporal location, and rate of recurrence of events in our everyday life" (Zerubavel, 1981, p. 14). In the psychologists' view, the coordinating process is one of cognitive and/or personality development. Some psychologists stress the dominance of the biological process and the significance of genetic factors in personality development (Freud, Eysenck). Eysenck states, following Royce and Powell, that there are personality traits that remain stable in life and find the explanation in inheritance. He claims that the general observation that genetic factors contribute between one-half and two-thirds of the phenotypic variance also applies to the stable personality traits (Eysenck, 1986, p. 217). He also supports a physiologically-based theory of personality (1986, p. 219). According to structuralists, such as Piaget and Levinson, the process of development creates and adapts a mental structure which mediates current behaviour and directs subsequent development. In Piaget's theory, the structure ("scheme") represents a person's view or knowledge of the world (cognitive structure) and enables the person to interact with that world (Miller, 1983, chapter 1). The structure proposed by Levinson and referred to as "life structure" is how a person views his life at a given time or, in Levinson's words, "the underlying pattern or design of a person's life at a given time" (1978, p. 41). The concept is related to the concept of personality (Levinson and Gooden, 1985, p. 5). The organization of the view of oneself and the world into structures and the adaptation of these structures take time. Because of this, we can identify stages in a person's life. Both Piaget and Levinson distinguish stable stages of structure-building (organization, consolidation) and unstable stages of transition from one structure to the next. In the transition periods, the life structure is reassessed and a new hierarchy of career processes is built.

In this paper, the coordinating process is assumed to interpret the various career orientations and the associated life goals, to assess the achievement along each career and to allocate resources (time, energy) to the career processes. Only processes that receive resources are active. The allocation mechanism determines the maximum speed of each process or, in case of symbiosis, the maximum speed of intertwined processes. External conditions cannot activate a process directly. They can, however, stimulate a process to demand the coordinating process for resources. This request will most likely initiate an assessment of "Where am I ?" (position-taking) by the coordinating process, involving the status of the other processes. Whether the request is granted depends on the result of the assessment. The coordinating process activates other processes and allocates resources but it cannot ensure that the active processes generate the desired outcomes (events). In order to produce a desired outcome, the context or situation must meet the process requirements. In other words, an active process produces an event only if the circumstances permit. For instance, a job search process results in a job if a suitable job is available.

A basic question is: What governs the coordinating process ? We adopt the view that the coordinating process is governed by career orientations, which are derived from life (developmental) goals, and by stimuli from the various career processes and from the environment. Of primary importance for the career orientations are the life goals rather than the role status determined by the social environment. The view that demographic behaviour is an expression of human development rather than role status is best formulated by Held: "Marriage and procreation may come to be seen merely as experiences of an exploring, growing self and no longer as role and status positions" (Held, 1986, p. 162). The impact of society on behaviour is mediated by the development process, which in Erikson's theory is the quest for identity. Norms do not affect behaviour directly, but affect the identity which in turn affects behaviour. The career orientations provide a meaning for the building of a life structure. The coordinating process assesses the messages it receives from the other processes and the environment, and designs an action scheme (career strategy). One scheme may be "wait", in which case the information received is kept in a buffer (memory) until the process is ready to act. The mental frame in which the messages are processed is itself an outcome of previous stimuli (learning mechanism). It is closely related to the scheme-concept of Piaget. In this view, external stimuli help to determine the development path. The design of a life structure is an adaptive mechanism to increase the ability to perform (survive) in the given environment and to achieve the life goals.

If the coordinating process functions properly, the life events follow an ordered sequence and the stages take long enough to create the developmental readiness for the next stage. In addition, the parallel careers advance in harmony and the life course is free of tension or stress.

2.7. Work and Family

2.7.1. The significance of career orientation

The life course perspective developed in this paper may be used to investigate the interdependence between work and family careers. Differences in observed career patterns may in part be explained in terms of differences in career orientations, i.e. in attitudes regarding the future life course. In the demographic literature, career orientation and personality traits in general are rarely used explicitly to explain behaviour over the life course. It is somewhat surprising given the popularity of attitudinal research (e.g. Fishbein model). There exist a few exceptions however. Bulatao and Fawcett (1981, p. 437) find that women with higher occupational aspirations are more likely to postpone early childbearing. Bernhardt relates labour force attachment of women to their basic orientation, which is "some kind of personality trait or attitudinal dimension" (Bernhardt, 1987, p. 2). She explains: "Family-oriented women regard paid work as something transitory and marriage and children as indispensable, while work-oriented women regard employment as a life goal and marriage and children as possibilities." (Bernhardt, 1987, p. 2). Other scholars at the University of Stockholm, Section of Demography, have used the notion of career orientation to explain behavioural patterns (Hoem and Hoem, 1989, p. 64; Korpi, 1989, p. 10). Regan and Roland (1985) adopt a similar perspective. Based on the position taken by Almquist *et al.* (1980) that women choose careers to complement lifestyle choices, they construct a lifestyle commitment variable with five categories: family-directed (family most important life goal, any other goal except work career second most important), family-accommodated (family most important life goal, career second most important), career-accommodated (career most important, family second most important), career-directed (career most important, any other goal except family second most important) and other-directed (neither family nor career as most important).

The existence of a career orientation partly explains the behavioural consistency over time, in particular the effect of early demographic behaviour on the later life course. This statement is supported by longitudinal research carried out by Mott and Shapiro (1983). Using data from the first ten years of the National Longitudinal Surveys of Labor Market Experience of Young Women (USA), the authors found that (i) the traditional pattern work - childbearing and -rearing - work has been eroding and that young women are choosing to retain close ties to the labour market during the months just before and even just after childbearing; and that (ii) early work behaviour has no effect on later fertility. Early employment is a good predictor of work attachment during the life course, however: "The strong link between early employment and later attachment to work has been documented and shown to be independent of inter- vening fertility." (Mott and Shapiro, 1983, p. 250). Nakamura and Nakamura (1984a) arrived at the same conclusion: "There is little evidence that a woman's child status, including the presence of a new baby, has any current effect on her work behaviour after controlling for her work behaviour in the previous year." (1984a, p. 23). As Bernhardt and others in Sweden and Holden (1983) in Japan, Mott and Shapiro rely on psychological factors to explain the finding:

> "We believe that work activity during the months surrounding the first birth reflects in large part an unmeasured 'commitment to work' that is operative in influencing work activity throughout the life cycle. Young women who remain employed until just before giving birth and who return to work shortly after the birth are regarded as manifesting greater motivation to work, or greater 'tastes' for market work. Their early work behaviour may well be reflecting longer-term aspects of a psychological 'need' for work activity, career satisfaction, and perhaps also a status based on activity outside the home." (Mott and Shapiro, 1983, pp. 250-251).

This view is consistent with Runyan's (1984, p. 212) assertion that the impact of early experience on the later life course is mediated by personality traits.

The concept of career orientation is a useful aid in causal analysis of life course events. The temporal ordering of behaviour is not a good indication of causality, since people think prospectively and anticipate events or conditions. This is particularly well illustrated in studies of the relation between employment and birth spacing. Coleman (1983) presents an interesting analysis of Japanese families. He shows how young married couples carefully try to space childbirths, not just with regard to present demand-and-supply factors in labour for infant care but also with a view to the husband's probable career advancement and thus the family's capacity a decade and more

in the future, to provide support for two or more offspring simultaneously in
college. This behaviour is fully consistent with a career strategy to achieve
life or developmental goals. The finding of Ni Bhrolchain (1986a, b) is equally
interesting. Using employment and fertility histories from two British longitudinal surveys, he tests Keyfitz's (1977, p. 329) proposition that work-
oriented women shorten their birth intervals to hasten the end of childbearing
and -rearing and thus to return to work (see also Sweet, 1973, pp. 118-120,
and Standing, 1978, p. 167). Women who do not anticipate paid employment would
prefer a well-spaced family and thus longer birth intervals. The analysis shows
that the proposition only applies to women who do not work between births. Ni
Bhrolchain therefore concludes that there are two employment effects on spacing
(1986b, p. 147): a positive effect associated with work during the interval
and a negative effect associated with speed of return after childbearing. The
two opposing effects are thought of as the influence of current and future
work, respectively. The significance of the current work orientations is
however dependent on the availability of child care, allowing women to work
between births. The finding that in the 1970s the increased engagement in
interbirth working did not significantly lengthen the birth intervals is very
interesting in this regard (1986b, p. 151). For a review of the literature on
the relation between employment and birth spacing, the reader is referred to
Ni Bhrolchain (1986a, pp. 65-66). The design of a career strategy involving
explicitly the timing of life events in relation to other events has been
referred to as "timetable consciousness." Plath (1983, p. 155) defines it as
the consideration of the present scheduling of life events on the remaining
career.

2.7.2. The significance of context

Career orientations are not the only factors shaping a person's life course.
The context in which a person operates is also important. The context determines the choice set or set of options among which the person may choose. In
this respect, Avioli's finding on the employment status of married women in
the USA is revealing: black employed wives are working out of financial needs,
while their white counterparts appear to be working not so much out of
financial need but rather out of an interest in being in the labour force
(Avioli, 1985, p. 744). White wives derive satisfaction from their labour force
status, while stress devolves to black wives. If the context in which a person

operates is demanding, the freedom of choice is limited and the effect of individual differences on behaviour will be reduced (Mischel, 1977). In that case, the consistency between attitudes-orientations and behaviour gradually disappears (Tazelaar, 1983, p. 119). The contextual or situational pressure should therefore be considered in life course studies. Many people may not have any choice at all; they can only select the most suitable adaptation to the constraints. But they may also try to change the context. The micro-context is shaped by the person as much as the life of the person is shaped by it. Marriage and migration are clear illustrations of how a person may influence the micro-context and hence the available career options. But the significance of other behavioural events may not be less. For instance, school drop-out severely restricts the employment career options. Prolonged education, on the other hand, increases the number of career options, everything else remaining constant. Analogously, being financially independent increases the freedom of choice of life goals and career strategies to achieve the goals.

There are numerous examples of the micro-context influencing the work behaviour of women. The attitude of family members has shown to significantly affect women's paid work involvement (Spitze, 1988). Another example, the availability of child care, flexible working hours and work in or around the home, affect women's labour force participation by removing a barrier to labour force entry and by reducing the incompatibility between work and children. Spitze (1988, p. 606) reports on research in the USA, which shows that approximately one out of six nonemployed women would look for employment if high-quality, affordable child care were available. In the Netherlands, it is one out of ten[2] (Wilbrink-Griffioen *et al.*, 1988, p. 138). The context, in particular the availability of child care, mediates the relation between fertility and employment.

The career orientation and the context (cultural, financial, facilities) in which a woman operates explain most of the interdependence between fertility and employment careers. But there are additional factors. One is career uncertainty. Few authors explicitly account for uncertainty. Greene and Quester (1982) found that the perceived risk of marital dissolution positively affects the work career attachment of women. This behaviour cannot be explained by the need for self-actualization, but by the need to protect oneself and the

---

[2] Included are women with at least one child under age four. About 75 per cent of these women are not engaged in paid work and about 30 per cent of these wish to engage in paid work.

children from economic deprivation. In order to understand the relation between career orientation and career behaviour, uncertainty must be taken into account.

Another factor is associated with the job or type of paid work. Jansweijer *et al.* (1988, p. 85) report an interesting finding: in the Netherlands, many women leave their job upon the birth of their first child, in particular if the prospects for promotion are not good. Job satisfaction and prospects therefore enter the decision to stay in employment or not after the birth of the first child. On the other hand, a woman may hold on to her job since leaving could put her at risk of not finding a suitable job when needed.

The interdependence between fertility and labour force participation of women in the West is characterized by the "combination strategy", a term introduced by Bernhardt (1987, p. 9). Women wishing to combine work and family careers have a limited number of options to choose from, all involving the provision of child care. Child care resolves part of the incompatibility of work and family careers. Presser (1986, 1988) finds that in the 1980s in the USA, about half of all care to children of employed mothers is provided by the parents or by relatives. For the Netherlands, the figure is 60 percent (Wilbrink-Griffioen *et al.*, 1988, p. 134). Of young dual-earner parents in the USA, one fourth are the principal providers of care when mothers are employed (Presser, 1988, p. 135). Spouses may select part-time employment and/or flexible working hours to share child care responsibilities. Close to one third of full-time workers and about two fifths of part-timers work other than fixed daytime schedules (Presser, 1988, p. 137). They may also involve relatives. One third of all care to children of employed mothers in the USA are given by relatives, mainly grandparents (Spitze, 1988, p. 607). Comparable figures are not available for the Netherlands. Shift work is likely to increase for two unrelated reasons. First, the growth in female employment is largely absorbed by the service sector, which has the highest proportion of shift workers among dual-earners couples.[3] Second, relatives (notably grandmothers) are becoming less available for child care with increasing geographical mobility and the increasing employment of older women (Presser, 1988, p. 147).

The options may also be affected by the past career. Korpi (1989, p. 19) suggests that increased work experience gives women a better opportunity to

---

[3] In the Netherlands, 85 per cent of all employed women have a job in the service sector (Jansweijer *et al.*, 1988, p. 81). Most employed women working flexible hours have children to take care of (Jansweijer *et al.*, 1988, p. 83).

realize the combination strategy because part-time jobs are easier to get for women with work experience.

2.8. Conclusion

Empirical research on the relationship between fertility and labour force participation of women did not result in consistent findings. One reason is the data used to identify the causal structure. Cross-sectional surveys, which provided most of the data in early studies, overestimate the interdependence between fertility and employment. It became clear that cross-sectional data cannot be used to study individual behaviour (Nakamura and Nakamura, 1985). Longitudinal data, which contain information on previous behaviour show a picture that differs considerably from the cross-section. Longitudinal studies reveal that early experience is a good predictor of subsequent behaviour. But how to explain the observations ? This paper aimed at contributing to the explanation by concentrating on process dynamics. Observed patterns of fertility and employment are outcomes of parallel career processes, which continuously interact with each other and with their common environment. In these particular career processes, the interaction is due to shared resources (time and energy). An individual has a limited amount of time and energy to allocate to family and work. Moreover, both careers are in their critical stages at about the same time. If the two careers are to be combined, the incompatibility needs to be resolved, either by appropriate scheduling of the life events (birth, labour market entry and exit) or by resources provided by others (by members of the support network or by the formal sector).

Although available longitudinal studies have increased our understanding of the interdependence between work and family careers substantially; they have an important shortcoming preventing a complete understanding of how career processes interact. The surveys focus on overt behaviour. But in most cases, behaviour is merely a manifestation of what goes on in a person's mind. In order to understand behavioural patterns, we need to identify and describe the mental processes, in particular the process of human development. Whether human development is governed by the quest for identity, as in Erikson's life course theory, by a process of adaptation to and assimilation of the social context, as in Piaget's theory, or even by a biological process is not of the greatest relevance at this stage of research. What is significant, however, is that behavioural patterns can only be understood if they can be related to the underlying processes that constitute the causal mechanism. In this paper, the causal link between behavioural patterns in different domains of life is associated with a coordinating process, an abstract construct that processes information, keeps time by comparing the actual development to an intrinsic standard and allocates resources. Interactions between processes within the individual and between the individual and the micro- and macro-context are mediated by the coordinating process. It therefore mediates behaviour and directs subsequent development.

How information is processed, time is kept and resources are allocated remains largely unknown, except for the circadian timing system in biology (Moore-Ede *et al.*, 1982). Developmental psychology provides some partial clues (Miller, 1983). In this paper, we attach significance to career orientations, which are derived from the quest to meet a hierarchy of needs and are part of the personality structure. Although the personality structure, and therefore also the career orientations, changes over time as a result of the process of personality development, the basic *predisposition* to develop certain traits remains stable. At this stage of research, the predisposition is believed to be genetically determined.

The existence of a predisposition to develop certain personality traits is the basis of behavioural consistency, which in turn explains why early experience remains a good predictor of subsequent behaviour and early behaviour a good predictor of the life course, keeping in mind that relations between factors are probabilistic and not deterministic. Early experience is, of course, not always an effect of predisposition; it can occur by accident. Once one goes down a path, the forces of circumstance and the progressive investment of time and energy work together to make one continue along it (Hoem and Hoem, 1989, p. 65).

An implication of the existence of a predisposition is selection. Persons who choose to work for pay and to go into certain jobs are different from persons who choose to stay at home to raise a family. Very recently, authors have come to rely on latent traits and the associated selectivity to explain differences in employment and fertility patterns (e.g. Mott and Shapiro, 1983, p. 250; Spitze, 1988, p. 610). The latent traits correspond to the unobserved heterogeneity, frequently referred to in statistical analyses of career transitions and providing an explanation for the empirical finding that the longer a person remains in a state or stage, the less likely he is to leave the state or stage (duration effect).

The impact of personality development on demographic behaviour is likely to grow. Self-actualization, the highest aspiration in Maslow's hierarchy of needs, is in reach of many and is becoming a norm for others. "The strong emphasis on individualism requires people to search constantly for guiding and stabilizing orientations, for an individual life style and a personal identity" (Van de Kaa, 1988, p. 21). But many will search in vain or will end in a lifetime of stress if incompatibilities between parallel careers are not resolved or the lower-level needs are not met. A better understanding of the complex interdependencies between parallel careers and the significance of personal differences in career orientations should contribute to the removal of the incompatibilities and other constraints on harmonious human development.

SOCIAL APPROVAL, FERTILITY AND FEMALE LABOUR MARKET[1]

Siegwart Lindenberg
Vakgroep Sociologie / ICS
Rijksuniversiteit Groningen
Grote Rozenstraat 31
9712 TG GRONINGEN
The Netherlands

3.1. Introduction

Maybe the most important development in the last thirty years with regard to theory formation in the social sciences is what with the help of hindsight can now be called "economic imperialism." (cf. Lindenberg, 1985) But while this may be true for theory formation, much of the substantive insights are to be found in the more messy social sciences, like anthropology and sociology. The economic approach to fertility and labour market behaviour does not seem to me to be an exception to this state of affairs. The most sophisticated models on the subject today are economic in origin (cf. overview Siegers, 1985 and especially Willis, 1973, Becker, 1981). But models only lead to substantive claims by the assumptions made concerning their parameters, what has been called "bridge assumptions" that bridge the distance between the model and reality, at least to some (hopefully increasing) degree. Becker's book (1981) for example, is full of bridge assumptions, but the most important one is also the one he is most proud of: that the relevant tradeoff in the decision to have children is quantity versus quality. This assumption helps solve the puzzle "that the demand for children is highly responsive to price and perhaps to income, even when children have no close substitutes." (Becker, 1981, p. 107).

There have been different kinds of criticism of this basic bridge assumption, but the most essential seems to me that it is not really an assumption connecting the model to reality (e.g. Witt, 1987; Van Horn, 1988). It is very plausible that the quality per child and the number of children are both important aspects for a couple, but there is little evidence that these

---

[1] Many people have contributed valuable suggestions towards the revision of this paper. I would like to thank the participants of the conference, and among them especially Jacques Siegers, for their valuable suggestions. Special thanks for close reading and constructive criticism also go to Peter van der Meer from the ICS at Groningen.

two dimensions are the ones most relevant for decision making, i.e. that the relevant trade-off is being made between these two. There are other ways of explaining the price responsiveness than quantity and quality, and they are closer to the social reality of the couple than the latter.

Yet another disadvantage of the New Home Economics approach has also been voiced before: the fact that it treats the couple as a unit rather than as two persons who have to consider each other's wishes in their decision making. As will be seen, the "social-production-function" approach taken here does consider this interaction prominently.

In this paper, I try to present some arguments for the reorientation of some bridge assumptions found in the economic approach to fertility and female labour market behaviour, especially the one about quantity and quality. The emphasis is on "reorientation" rather than on presenting a fully-fledged theory of fertility and female labour market behaviour. For example, I will not go into questions of helping children on farms or the role of children for the security of the parents' old age.

3.2. Constraint-centered heuristic, general human goals and social production functions

One way to "sociologize" economic model building is to do what economists generally leave undone, namely to explain preferences and preference changes (in the sense of change of taste or values). Andorka, at the end of his famous overview of work done on determinants of fertility, says: "without better knowledge of these preferences, the economic theory of fertility seems to miss the most important factors determining long-term changes in fertility in advanced countries" and sociologists would have to supply this better knowledge (Andorka, 1978, p. 383). A similar point has variously been made about micro-economics in general, for example by Von Weizsäcker (1984) and Opp (1985b). Good advice ?

We have a hundred years of experience with a preference-centered heuristics in sociology and I can only advise against it on the basis of the accumulated experience in that field. A preference-centered heuristics will drive out detailed attention to constraints, such as price and income changes. Worse yet, a preference-centered heuristics will draw increasingly more attention to situations that influence values held by people, i.e. to social-

ization episodes, drawing attention away from choice because constraints (i.e.
alternatives) play virtually no explanatory role. We know from traditional
sociology, in which behaviour has been explained by values, that the concepts
of choice, scarcity, and constraints have had no place, which is what makes
it so difficult to relate the empirical insights on the gender division of
labour, on the interaction in the family, on labour market behaviour etc.
(mostly couched in "role" terms) to theoretical models.

There is another, and I think better, way of sociologizing economic model
building, and that is by assuming that virtually all goods are means with the
exception of a very few. If we assume some general human goals, identical for
everybody, as Stigler and Becker (1977) did, then also indifference curves turn
into constraints, namely functions related to the production of the general
human goals. In this way we would have a constraint-driven heuristics, and if
we stick our necks out (unlike Stigler and Becker) and name the general human
goals, then the heuristics cannot be shifted in an ad hoc manner from
constraint to preference heuristics and back. The most prominent candiates for
a list of general human goals in the general discussion on such goals are
physical well-being and *social approval* (see Lindenberg, 1984). There may be
others, but the list will be short and "children" are very likely not on it.

It is obvious that his kind of constraints heuristics is oriented towards
production rather than consumption, similar to the New Home Economics. But now
that the two general goals have been named, the *basic questions* about individuals in society to be asked are: *how can this individual systematically
produce physical well-being* and *how can he or she systematically produce social
approval* ? The answers to these two questions may not be very precise, but they
will convey, even in rough outline, the most fundamental elements of social
structure. Elsewhere, I have called them "social production functions"
(Lindenberg, 1984).

A refinement of this approach is to distinguish some different forms of
social approval which, up to a point, can be substituted for one another (cf.
Lindenberg, 1986). In this paper, I will make considerable use of this
refinement.

3.3. Status, behavioural confirmation and affect

A phenomenological study of the various forms of social approval would have
to make fine distinctions, but for my purposes here it is enough to work with
rougher categories. I distinguish between three kinds of social approval:
status, behavioural confirmation, and positive affect. Since all three are
relational, I, for the purpose of discussion, will make use of two fictitious
interaction partners, viz. Ego and Alter.

Status is social approval given on the basis of the *relative* command over
scarce goods such as privilege, money, extraordinary talent, power, influence,
certain kinds of knowledge, luxury goods, etc. The amount of status from the
command of such goods depends on the distribution of these goods, thus status
distinguishes people relative to each other (this is called a "positional"
good).

Being positively distinguished from others on some valued dimension is
clearly rewarding for human beings. Status can be produced by things Ego does
or acquires. What these things are depends on the times and on the particular
society. For the present-day Western societies, obvious examples are getting
an education, working for and getting high political office, acquiring
conspicuous consumption goods. At the same time, status may also be produced
by things Ego has been given (without any additional effort or other costs on
her part). What these things are depends again on the times and the particular
society. Examples from the past are privileges given at birth and status-
conferring titles.

Behavioural confirmation is the feeling to have done "the right thing"
in the eyes of relevant others. Having one's expectations met is rewarding
which, in turn, elicits a positive response. In other words, when Alter's
behavioural expectation vis-à-vis Ego in a face-to-face situation is met, Alter
will give off a verbal or nonverbal response indicating to Ego that she has
done it right. If Ego is not convinced of the opposite, she will accept Alter's
response as a behavioural confirmation. When Alter's reaction can be easily
and accurately predicted, Ego can experience behavioural confirmation even in
Alter's absence. Under such circumstances, Ego can pat herself on the back for
having done something "right", but without frequent confirmation by others,
predicting their reactions will become difficult and thus anticipatory self-
praise will also become less likely.

Expectations can be personal or shared. Relatively stable expectations (regarding a certain kind of behaviour in a certain kind of recurring situation) shared between at least two persons are called "social norms" in sociology. Everybody is part of at least one social circle and in this circle there are at least some recurring situations subject to norms shared by the members of the circle. Over time, these norms will have produced more or less repetitive, norm-conform behaviour which, in turn, keeps creating behavioural confirmation as a by-product. In this sense, everybody has a certain endowment with behavioural confirmation, but the size of the endowment can vary considerably.

Of course, Ego can also attempt to produce confirmation directly where norms permit laudable, extraordinary ways of conformity; or she can attempt to meet the personal expectations of certain relevant others; she can also join social circles with more norms and purposefully try to meet all expectations, maybe even in the hope of building up routinized, norm-conform behaviour and thus endowment with confirmation. In short, Ego can also invest in goods for the production of behavioural confirmation.

Positive affect is what Ego gets from Alter if Ego and Alter are involved in an affective relationship. A central ingredient in such a relationship is that Ego and Alter care for each other. "Caring for somebody" here means that indicators of Ego's utility have become goods which produce a certain amount of physical well-being in Alter and vice versa.

While the exact psychological causes of positive affect (in the sense used here) are not yet well explored (cf. Rubin, 1973), it is known that three conditions will jointly produce and affective relationship: the more valuable Ego's transfers or externalities for Alter and vice versa; the more Ego meets the behavioural expectations of Alter and vice versa; and the more Ego and Alter interact informally on a continuous basis. In contrast to behavioural confirmation, positive affect is always personal.

It is also possible to purposefully create the conditions that produce positive affect. For example, given frequent interaction and positive externalities of Alter on Ego, Ego can try to please Alter by positive transfers (attention, gifts, helping, etc.) and doing what she thinks Alter expects of her.

If we look at all three components of social approval, we see that only status is a positional good (see Hirsch, 1978). It is by definition not possible that everybody gets a high status, since status is based on the relative difference between people. By contrast, behavioural confirmation and positive affect could in principle be evenly distributed throughout the society. For this very reason, these two goods are particularly important sources of social approval for people with a low status endowment.

3.4. The fundamental exchange

Given physical well-being and social approval as general human goals, the question arises what the basic social production functions with regard to our topic at hand are. As a basis for arriving at the rough outlines of the relevant social production functions, I would like to start with what may be called the *fundamental exchange*. The idea of a basic exchange has often been formulated, it is also assumed in Becker's *A Treatise on the Family* (1981), and it rests on two assumptions:

a.   a "home" is of fundamental importance for the production of physical well-being;

b.   with the exception of some complementary activities, there are gains from specialization in "making a home" and in "providing the means for making a home", leading to a division of labour among the specialists.

The fundamental exchange is the exchange between the specialists: "making a home" in exchange for "providing the means for making a home" and vice versa. Added to the usual reasons for gains from specialization, I should mention two important extra points: the effect of patterns of attention (framing) on the execution of tasks (Lindenberg, 1989) and the importance of separate spheres of competence for mutual social approval of close partners (De Vries, 1988). Both effects would make gains from specialization likely even if the human capital and the labour market position of the partners were identical (which, in all likelihood, they are not).

The assumption that at all times the specialists for "making a home" are far more frequently to be found among the women than among the men has been much criticized as being ideological (e.g. Rogers, 1980) and yet the evidence against it seems to be even weaker than the evidence for it. In any case, I will make this assumption. I will not go into detail in analysing what goes into "making use of a home", for this category is a container for many different activities (including eating, sleeping, sex), but it is clear that with increasing income it will be possible to make a home that will provide higher levels of physical well-being.

On the basis of the foregoing discussion we can now specify part of the social production function for physical well-being. For men it contains "providing the means for making a home" and "making use of the home"; and for women, it contains "making use of the means provided for making a home", "making a home" and "making use of the home." In the socio-biological literature there is some evidence for the assumption of "kin altruism." For this reason, I will include "children" in the social production function of physical well-being for both men and women. Since affective relationships need continuous informal interaction to develop and maintain, children would not yield positive affect without a home. For this reason, men and women would first have a home before they would decide on having children.

In sociology and cultural anthropology, the gender related division of labour has often been described and discussed. And probably most of the empirical work on describing behaviour and attitudes of males and females in households comes from these studies. In theoretical terms, Parsons (1954), inspired by the group psychology of Bales, has provided the "pattern" of discussion by viewing the family as a universal nuclear group with one "instrumental" (male) and one "expressive" (female) leader, socializing children into the respective roles for adult life. Typical questions within sociology have focussed on these role assignments; for example: Are they changing over time ? Can they be weakened by adult socialization ? Can they conflict with other roles ? (e.g. Berger and Wright, 1978; Bernard, 1981).

There are some similarities between the role-theoretical approach and the social-production-function theory. Both the gender roles and the fundamental exchange are gender allocations of tasks, and interpreted as normative expectations, roles are means for reaching social approval in exchange for conformity. They can thus be part of a social production function. A crucial difference, however, between the two is this: roles will change when people are taught differently, and thus presumably the gender division of labour is a matter of cultural inertia to be brought to a halt and reversed if there is an emancipatory movement of sufficient strength. The approach taken here comes to another conclusion: roles reflect the factual division of labour in a previous period. Propaganda for different role expectations will have some effect (via the reduction of behavioural confirmation of standard role behaviour due to the controversy over norms) but it will not undo or even reverse the role expectations if it does not undo or reverse the gains from specialization in the fundamental exchange. Yet, gains from specialization are no part and (due to the difference in implied action theories) cannot be part of role theory. For this paper, there is yet another difference even more important: in combination with a reasonable theory of action, the social-production-function theory can be used to explain a great deal of phenomena observed by sociologists, including action that deviates from the role pattern.

3.5. Elements of a theory of fertility and female labour market behaviour

So far, we have some important elements of the social production functions for physical well-being. Next, we establish some elements for the production functions for social approval in its three different forms. Due to the fact that social approval can only be given if it is generally known when to give it, the following assumptions are quite commonsensical.

Status
In Western societies, there are two major sources of status: somebody's *occupation* in society at large and his or her *life style*. While Max Weber (1921/1958) may have been the first to analyse the status features of life styles systematically, it had long been the subject of literary treatment. Similarly, the ordering of occupations according to prestige has been measured and described by sociologists and it is, by its very nature, generally recognized. Of course there are also minor sources of status, such as stratified positions in voluntary organizations. In a more extended version of the theory, these sources would certainly have to be included, but here they will be ignored.

Behavioural Confirmation
The rewarding aspect about behavioural confirmation is the indication by others (and by oneself) that one has "done something right." If there are no clear expectations, there will be no such reward and if the expectations differ from one person to the next, there will be much less reward accumulating than if something is "generally expected and met with approval." As stated above, such general expectations are only produced by social norms which have the added

advantage that the person can reward herself in anticipation of the predictable response of others.

Positive Affect

Again, in Western societies, there are two major sources of affect: a relationship with one's own children (and parents), and a relationship with a life-sharing partner. In many families, parents and children interact informally on a continuous basis. On the basis of socio-biological reasoning, we assume that parents care for their children which means they are willing to put themselves out for their children (with net positive transfers). In addition, parents meet many of the expectations of their children and the children are taught to fulfill the behavioural expectations of the parents (socialization). Thus the conditions for the development of an affective relationship between parents and children are likely to be met. The same holds true for adults who live together, frequently reward each other without any immediate quid pro quo and often meet each other's expectations. Of course there are also minor sources of affect, such as friends, pets and valued objects (e.g. cars). In a more extended version of the theory, these sources would have to be included, but here they will be ignored.

Let us now take a representative "traditional" couple and look at the rough outlines of their social production functions. For the man, "making use of the home", "providing the means for making a home" and "children" are all part of the social production functions for physical well-being. But given the fundamental exchange, "providing the means for making a home" is *the* way for the man to produce physical well-being and for reasons of efficiency he will attempt to combine this production with the production of status via occupational prestige. Another way of saying this is that he will seek an optimal combination of income and status rather than go for the highest paying job or the most prestigious occupation without concern for the other. Similarly, he will attempt to combine "making use of the home" and "having children" with gaining status from his "life style." In other words, he will leave "creating a life style" as much as possible to his wife. Thus he depends for his physical well-being and for part of his status on the activities of his wife. To the degree that the activities surrounding occupation and life style are both governed by social norms, he will be able to gain behavioural confirmation from both. His affect can come from his relationship with his wife and/or from children.

The fundamental exchange makes it expedient for the wife to combine "making a home and using the means provided" with "creating a life style." Since there is no special status for "creating" versus "having" a particular life style and since the wife has no occupational prestige, the wife has less status than the husband. One way to increase the total of her social approval is to increase her affect by having children, and presumably the more children, the more affect. This possibility of increasing social approval is constrained by her ability to combine having children with making a home and creating a life style and by the affective needs of her husband. To a considerable degree, the number of children may define the range of life styles. Then again, the more the activities surrounding making a home, having children and living a particular life style are governed by social norms, the more the wife gains behavioural confirmation from all three.

The first testable hypothesis concerns the strength of the fundamental exchange, and it is derived from the idea that "making a home" is the more clearly defined the more it *also could* accommodate offspring.

> *(H1)* The more a man and a woman are socially defined as a couple which is in a social position to procreate, the stronger the fundamental exchange will operate when they form a home together.

Thus, in most Western societies, the fundamental exchange should be stronger for a married couple than for an unmarried couple that lives together.

The other testable hypotheses generated by the theory and considered in this paper fall into four groups: first, those related to the barrier effect against changing the social production function; second, those related to potential threats to the fundamental exchange; third, those related to the source social approval; and fourth, the hypotheses concerning change in number of children, life-style, partner relationship and work.

3.5.1. Changes in social production functions

Our representative couple has the elements of "traditional" social production functions: *he* provides, shares in the life style and enjoys his occupational status; *she* makes the home, creates the life style and has children. The basic elements in social production functions are tied to human capital accumulations and a way of life, so that changes can be quite traumatic.

Regarding the difficulty of the hurdle that has to be taken, it is useful to distinguish three kinds of changes: those that are normatively expected and are thus supposed to happen, those that are not supposed to happen, and those that may or may not happen. Growing up entails normatively expected changes in social production functions, and there are other such life cycle changes as marriage, having the first child and retirement. The point is that normatively expected changes are eased by anticipatory socialization and by behavioural confirmation, while unexpected ones are more costly and normatively disallowed changes are almost prohibitive. Clearly, ideological publicity work (such as to be found in the women's movement) can slowly reduce that price because of their effect on attitudes. But against the role-theoretic prediction concerning this point, I would assume that even changed attitudes will not affect the fundamental exchange and its workings. Skeen *et al.* (1989), working within a role-theoretic framework when comparing American, Brazilian and Filippino attitudes towards the mother's work outside the home, state with some surprise that "there is still a universal acceptance of specified roles for men and women" and their role-theoretic expectations do no help them much to interpret the results. The social-production-function arguments made above can be stated in the following *hypotheses*:

> *(H2)* Working outside the home (no matter how few the hours per week) is a basic change in the social production function for those women who have not worked before they entered marriage and will therefore be more costly.

> *(H3)* To the degree that marriage is postponed and/or the first partnership is expressively not intended to be marriage-like, to that degree the likelihood that women will have worked before marriage will go up and thus the price of changing the social production function will go down.

Still crossovers are not unproblematical as the next section will discuss.

3.5.2. The impact of threats to the fundamental exchange

Theoretically, it is possible to say that when the husband cannot provide for making a home, the wife will also seek gainful employment. However, it is by no means clear at what point his income is "not enough." The husband may feel his home generates very little physical well-being, or the wife may feel that the task of making a home is impossible given the resources. Still, the income must be very low in order to render a home virtually impossible. Above that limit, it is likely that aspects of social approval play an important role again. Both the husband and the wife gain status (and to some degree behavioural confirmation) from their joint life style. But the wife has no other source of status and will thus be even more keen on keeping up some standard of life style. Thus, in all likelihood, she will want to enter gainful employment more than he would want her to.

This aspect is important because given the fundamental exchange, the husband has *a legitimate claim to the wife's time*. Every hour a wife is giving to an activity outside the home is subject to a legitimation check regarding the fundamental exchange. Serious conflict will arise if the wife crosses over into gainful employment when the husband does not agree. Why should he not agree ? He cannot have it both ways and keep his wife to the bargain without keeping his. When she says she has to go out and earn some money for making the home, she says, in effect, that he does not keep up the fundamental exchange, thereby forfeiting his claim to and basis for physical well-being. Letting her easily go to work outside would thus undermine his social production function. Stated as *hypotheses*:

(*H4*) The stronger the fundamental exchange, the more likely that the wife will work outside the home only in agreement with her husband.

(*H5*) The chance that a wife would work outside the home is the smaller, the more her doing so would threaten the fundamental exchange.

(*H6*) The chance that a husband would feel the fundamental exchange threatened by his wife's working outside the home increases with the strength of the fundamental exchange, number of young children the wife has and the number of hours she works.

Thus we expect that the stronger the fundamental exchange, the more likely that the wife will not work at all when having small children and work only part time otherwise, if she works at all.

> *(H7)* Given the expressed goal of the wife wanting to work outside the home for adding to the income that is needed to make a home, the husband will agree only grudgingly, withdrawing his agreement in pieces according to increases in his income. In other words, the wife's weekly hours of paid work will be highly negatively responsive to husband's income.

It is interesting to note that the wife also guards the fundamental exchange. This can be gleaned from the fact that the wife's estimation of how much the husband does in the house is regularly lower than the husband's estimation of his own contribution. This is especially true of couples where the wife does not work outside (cf. McKenry *et al.*, 1986; Berger-Schmitt, 1986).

It is quite a different matter when the fundamental exchange is not endangered by the wife's work outside. Since the legitimation check still holds, so does the hypothesis that the wife will only work outside the home in agreement with the husband and only within the confines of the fundamental exchange. However:

> *(H8)* When the fundamental exchange is not threatened, i.e. when the "provider" part is not in doubt, then the husband's agreement will be given much more easily than when it is in doubt. Then the wife's weekly hours of paid work will not be very responsive to husband's income.

Why would a wife like to work if the husband brings home "enough" money ? Because more money is always better ? I will turn to this question in a moment. But before that it should be stated that even if she wants to work, she will be confronted with a labour market that also considers the fundamental exchange to be operative.

> *(H9)* The potential employers will assume that a husband has a legitimate claim to his wife's time, potentially ending or reducing

a wife's employment commitment, so that the expected return on training and career costs invested in the wife will be statistically lower that invested in the husband.

(H10) A woman not married will have a high probability of marrying at some point and will therefore also (albeit to a lesser extent) be confronted with employers' expectations of a comparatively lower return on training and career costs invested in her.

These two hypotheses jointly imply statistical discrimination against women, the more so the more commitment the occupation in question requires.

3.5.3. Trade-offs in social approval and children

We have assumed that some degree of physical well-being and some degree of every form of social approval is necessary for the production of utility. However, there is also considerable room for trade-offs and substitution. For example, investing in the gain of occupational prestige may be more efficient than investing in the creation of more affect (say by having another child). For somebody else, with low schooling and little hope for improving his occupational prestige, the reverse may be true.

Imagine, making a home brings less behavioural confirmation for the wife. How would the wife react ? Would she have more children in order to compensate in affect what was lost in behavioural confirmation ? This is unlikely, because children would tie her even more to making a home while these activities do not bring much behavioural confirmation. Having more children may also clash with the life style that brings the most status and the ensuing reduction in status may not be outweighed by the loss of affect. Instead, she may look for behavioural confirmation and maybe some status elsewhere, namely in the world of paid work where both can still be had to some degree. *Because* she would not work in order to earn money, the husband will agree more readily and he may even be glad for the extra income that does not threaten the fundamental exchange and yet could be used to improve the life style (and thereby status), possibly (over-)compensating the cost of reduced time input of the wife in making a home. Time and again it had been shown that where husbands earn a decent living, women would like to work mainly for "social" reasons. For example, in a recent study on highly educated working mothers, Van Vonderen

(1987, pp.12 ff.) found again an overwhelming majority of non-monetary reasons, such as approval, social contacts, self-actualization, for working. This is, of course, different from pure volunteer work, because the combination of job (money) and occupation (status) by the husband has given pay a symbolic meaning of valuation of an activity that becomes an integral part of working for aspects of social approval. Yet, the money can be less than for the "provider", because the importance of non-monetary aspects of the job (also present for the husband) is made salient by the fundamental exchange that states that the woman is not the provider. Summarized in form of a *hypothesis*:

> *(H11)* The higher the husband's income, the more likely that the wife would work for less than her reservation wage (i.e. the wage she would ask if she worked solely for money), if she would work at all and if the job offers behavioural confirmation and some status related to her human capital.

For Becker (1981) and much of the New Home Economics, children are like durable goods without close substitutes, so that the price elasticity of children becomes a puzzle unless one distinguishes aspects of children (quantity and quality) as substitutes. The approach taken here is different from (and yet even closer to the production paradigm of) the New Home Economics: children are here taken to be a factor good for the production of *social approval*. Increasing prices for this good will create shifts in demand also of other factor goods (like goods that produce behavioural confirmation and goods that produce status). Yet, it is likely that the number of children will show some lumpiness. As stated in the following hypothesis, for reasons of similarity effects on the production of affect, two children are more likely than one if there are any.

It is well known that similarity in important dimensions increases the likelihood that positive affect develops between people, given close contact.

> *(H12)* The more similar a child to a parent genetically (i.e. in looks, traits and sex), the more likely that there will develop a relationship with positive affect between them, given close contact.

Thus, we expect that a couple wishes to have at least one child of each sex for reasons of the production of affect, if they want to have children at all. The most likely other source for the production of positive affect is the partner, and here again, similarity will play an important role.

(H13) The more similar the partners in education and status, the more likely that there will develop a relationship with positive affect between them, given close contact.

It is also well known that education affects close contact between partners:

(H14) The higher and the more similar the education of both partners, the more likely that they will have close contact.

In other words, we expect that the affective relationship between husband and wife, if it develops, will reduce the importance of children for the production of affect, and we expect this effect to occur more frequently with couples where both are highly educated than where only one or even none is highly educated. Thus:

(H15) The higher and the more similar the education of both partners, ceteris paribus, the more likely that they will have fewer children.

The affective relationship between partners will also affect the impact exerted by the fundamental exchange on their behaviour:

(H16) The more affective the relationship between the partners, the more likely that they will attempt to respect each other's wishes.

This hypothesis entails that the fundamental exchange will become weaker the stronger the affective tie between the partners and the more the wishes of at least one partner deviate from the fundamental exchange. For example, if the wife wants to work, then the husband will agree more easily when his relationship to his wife is affective than when it is not. If the wife wants her partner to increase his share in "making the home", then the likelihood that he will do so increases with the affectiveness of their relationship. This aspect will play an important role in the following scenario of change.

3.6. A scenario of change

The following scenario can be thought of as a verbal description of interrelated price changes that could eventually be modelled formally. The scenario
that would bring about a slow but definite sea change in the way the fundamental exchange works out is as follows.

Due to some cause (to be explained later), social norms in the family and
in the community become less and less pronounced. This would have as a consequence the reduction of behavioural confirmation in making a home and in life
style. Due to some other cause (to be explained later), the status attached
to a life style that can be produced together with making a home decreases.
This would reduce the only source of status for the woman and one of the
sources of status for the man. The person most highly affected on both counts
is the wife. What can she do ? The marginal effect of extra children on the
production of affection depends on the number she already has. If that number
is very low, say one, she would gain much affection by having another one. But
more likely, she has already three or four children and has to decide whether
to shift resources from the next (planned) child to the most obvious alternative: a status enhancing life style, i.e. one that is not completely a by-
product of making a home. Since the husband also lost a source of status (the
"by-product-life-style"), he is likely to agree to this shift of resources.
In the aggregate we would already observe a reduction in fertility. Let this
continue for some time.

With the reduction of children, and the reduction of social norms that
give behavioural confirmation to sex-segregated activity in home and community,
the adult partnership itself will be utilized as a source of affect. The
partners will share more time together and, in connection with a life style
that is not a by-product of making a home, i.e. with "going out" and doing
things outside the home, their need for affect outside their relation will be
further reduced, leading to a further shift of resources from children to the
life style, thereby reducing again the number of children. The increasing
importance of an outside life style may prominently include such aspects as
"female beauty", an aspect that also clashes with having many children.

Far from eliminating the fundamental exchange through an affective and
egalitarian relationship between the partners, this development may even
strengthen the fundamental exchange by bolstering the workings of consensus

within the partnership. The wife would not go out and work for pay if the husband was strongly against it.

The very changes that brought about this scenario also increased the importance of paid work for behavioural confirmation and status, especially for the woman. It is assumed that she would first work within the given (traditional) social production functions that do not contain paid work. Thus she would reduce the number of children, shifting resources to life style and having a more affectionate relationship with her husband. But as the same causes keep working, these shifts will not compensate the weight of the lost behavioural confirmation and status, and a changed social production function, which includes paid work, becomes more and more attractive for the production of exactly these goods. The question is, what is behind the slow moving sea change ?

3.7. The privatization in consumption

In a nutshell, the sea change is brought about by privatization in consumption which in turn is driven by increasing disposable income and public goods. Elsewhere, I have argued this process in some detail (Lindenberg, 1984 and 1986). Here, I will follow closely some parts of the 1986 article on privatization in consumption. Summarized, the argument runs as follows. *Sharing groups* (akin to clubs in the theory of clubs) are the main source of social norms in the sphere of and around the home and they tend to vanish with increasing disposable income and public goods. And the increasing level of welfare reduces the "specialness" of given life styles, thus reducing the status they wield. Let us look at the argument in some more detail.

3.7.1. Sharing Groups

Private goods and public goods are only the extremes of a continuum, with most goods being somewhere inbetween. Most every-day goods can be more or less private in consumption. For example, a family may share one' bathroom or may enjoy the luxury of one bathroom per person in which case the good has been completely privatized. Informal groups come into being on the basis of sharing the costs of those goods that none of the members could afford to purchase or produce alone. Thus, in informal groups, both consumption and costs are shared.

For example, a number of farmers in a village may share a combine-harvester, which none of them could afford as a private good. In the same village, farmers may share risks by sharing the costs of strokes of individual bad luck (such as illness).

Cost sharing (including sharing in production) means positive external-ities mutually exerted on one another. Everybody profits from the arrangement because everybody is able to consume a good she would have otherwise been too poor to have access to. The more goods are shared, ceteris paribus, the larger the mutual positive externalities. But *sharing in consumption* creates negative externalities. For example, one farmer would like to use the combine just when it is another farmer's turn to use it. Or the other's negligence causes the combine to be out on repair for a week.

3.7.2. The production of norms in social life

Rules serve many functions but two particular ones are especially important in our context: they are needed in order to establish and maintain social norms. As we have said above, social norms are relatively stable expectations (regarding a certain kind of behaviour in a certain kind of recurring situation) shared between at least two persons. Sharing may be the most important source of norm production and maintenance in social life. Given positive externalities and the opportunity for face-to-face interaction, a sharing group has to find ways to mitigate the negative externalities caused by sharing. At the basis, it will be in everybody's interest to come to agreements concerning terms of consumption, handling, maintenance responsibi-lities, etc. Thus the process of establishing these agreements is actually the process of establishing the sharing group (with difficulties in agreement resulting either in the exclusion of some potential members or in a complete failure of the establishment of the group). The importance of agreement on the terms of sharing will subsequently drive a whole *process of norm production* (or norm mobilization, if the norms are already established through other sharing arrangements). Very likely, this process will be facilitated by norm-entrepreneurs who (in return for extra social approval) will coordinate the norm production process. First of all, the agreements will be translated into behavioural rules that regulate sharing behaviour. Such rules can be used as standards against which behaviour is judged and they can be used for socializing new members into the existing arrangement.

Since it is in everybody's interest that the others keep to the sharing rules and since everybody has some temptation not to keep to these rules at all times, social norms on the importance of keeping to agreements (cf. Ullmann-Margalit, 1977; Opp, 1985b) and on reciprocity (which is the normative translation of the fact that the group depends on the maintenance of positive externalities) will develop next. These norms are hierarchically higher than the rules that regulate sharing of a particular good because they abstract from any particular sharing arrangement. They help to simplify the interpretation of deviations from lower order rules by preventing that deviations are seen as continued attempts at renegotiation of the terms of sharing. This step is absolutely essential for the joint production of a new shared good: a sanctioning system that provides the selective incentives for keeping to the lower level rules (cf. Yamagishi, 1986). Such a system consists of yet another layer of social norms in the hierarchy: norms on reacting approvingly and disapprovingly to positive and negative deviations, respectively; norms on procedures and the distribution of rights to interpret ambiguous situations with regard to existing norms (including norms on resolving conflicts); and norms on procedures and the distribution of rights to adapt the sanctioning system with regard to sanctions and sanctioning agents. Finally, due to changes in technology or income, the existing sharing arrangements may not remain advantageous for all or part of the group members. As a result, norms on procedures and the distribution of rights for changing the sharing arrangement and the rules based on them will emerge.

Since everybody has an interest in the emergence (or mobilization) of the norms at these various levels, everybody is interested in keeping transaction costs for the production of norms low. For this reason, there is a consensus on the importance of shared values that help coordinate the joint production of norms. Norm entrepreneurs will thus find it not just useful to dramatize shared values in the group, they will also find a general willingness to stress communality in values rather than differences. Daily life thus can be shot through and through with norms on various levels and with rituals for the dramatization of shared values. What will increase or decrease this importance of norms ?

3.7.3. Determinants of the importance of norms in social life

As we have seen, in the view taken here, it is not values that generate norms (as often assumed in sociology) but the consensus on the importance of norms that draws out communalities for the dramatization as common values. As a consequence, if the consensus on the importance of norms vanishes, then the common values will not keep the norm hierarchy from fading or crumbling. What then governs the pervasiveness of norms ? Two conditions are particularly important for the ease with which norms can develop and be maintained. First, the amount of goods that are being shared in daily life, and second, the size of the group.

The more goods are shared, the more attention will be paid to the entire hiearchy of norms in the group because this hierarchy stabilizes very different sharing arrangements; transaction and enforcement costs for lower level agreements and rules will be lower to the degree that members generally accept the higher order norms. Paying attention to higher order norms also means that members find it worth-while to take the effort to sanction violators and to put some effort into socializing newcomers (for instance children) into acceptance of these norms.

Second, since the norm hierarchy regulates cooperation in mixed-motive games, at least some individuals of the sharing group will have an incentive to violate the norms in any particular situation. Since we are talking about a face-to-face interacting group, the group will never be so big that norm violators can hide effectively. The relevant question is, therefore, not whether people can secretly violate the norms but whether people can undermine the existing norms with situational ad hoc agreements. The principle that is operative with regard to *negotiated deviations* is based on the fact that social norms are not just rules but established patterns of expectations, and it may be called *the veto principle*: given a set of norms that governs a particular situation, each person has veto power against an ad hoc agreement among the others to deviate from the norm. The larger the group, the more likely that at least one person is present who would not like to deviate from the norm. And since that person has veto power, the adherence to norms becomes more stable as the group size increases (within the boundary of a face-to-face interacting group). For example, let us assume that there is a norm to celebrate Christmas in a certain fashion. Let us also assume that this particular year, neither the husband nor the wife are much motivated to go through this celebration. If nobody else is present, they may quickly reach an agreement to skip the celebration this year. If however, a child or an aunt or friend would have been present who would have insisted on celebrating Christmas, this third person does not have to be powerful or persuasive to get the whole group to celebrate Christmas. The veto principle would have shifted the coordination back to the normative expectations. Like the gains from specialization discussed above, the veto principle is likely to depend on framing effects which are not captured by the standard versions of utility theory (cf. Lindenberg, 1989). In sum, the larger the sharing group, ceteris paribus, the more likely that the existing norm hierarchy will stay operative.

3.7.4. Endowments

The upshot of the discussion so far was that the more goods are being shared and the bigger the sharing group, the more attention is being paid to norms in following them, in sanctioning others and in socializing newcomers. It is easy to see that the more attention is being paid to norms, the more other people will routinely react evaluatively to one's behaviour in terms of its relation to norms. Since these norms enhance the weight of the *positive* externalities among the members of the group, there will be positive reactions to norm-conformity, not just negative reactions to deviance. In addition, under such circumstances, it is easy to reward oneself for norm-conformity in anticipation of other people's reactions. In terms of our discussion of forms of social approval, we can thus say that the more attention is being paid to norms, the more *behavioural confirmation* is being produced as a side effect of every day behaviour. Of course one can and will make extra efforts to get people to see that one followed (or even positively deviated from) the norm, in order to get behavioural confirmation. But the bulk of behavioural confirmation will come as a *by-product* of daily behaviour, the more so, the more attention is being paid to norms. This means that under these circumstances, people will be *endowed* with behavioural confirmation. Since the production of positive affect depends in part also on behavioural confirmation, it too will be a by-product, given the additional requirements of close interaction and positive transfers.

If for some reason the number of goods being shared were to decrease and the sharing group were to get smaller, the endowment with behavioural confirmation and with positive affect would clearly also decrease. We have seen how important changes in the endowment with behavioural confirmation and positive affect are likely to be for fertility and female labour market behaviour. The important question then is: under what circumstances do sharing arrangements change such that fewer goods are being shared and sharing groups become smaller ?

3.7.5. Change in sharing groups with increasing income

Using reasonable model assumptions, it can be shown (cf. Lindenberg, 1982) that increasing disposable income for any individual will generally decrease the size of the sharing group(s) of which this individual is a member. In other words, increase in disposable income per individual will increase privatization in consumption. *But this is a process over time*. It is not captured by cross-sectional comparison of incomes because the main effect runs via changes in the surrounding social structure (the endowment).

Briefly summarized, the argument runs as follows. Assuming individuals can come to a sharing agreement at all, there will be an optimal group size for each participant, depending on the individual's preference for the good, her income, the total price of the good, and the amount of negative externalities created by the sharing situations. If one person is added to the sharing group, the cost per person will go down (gain) but the negative externalities facing each individual will increase (loss). If the marginal gain equals the marginal loss, the sharing group will have reached its optimal size. Obviously, if one of the parameters changes, the optimal group size will also change. For example, if ten farmers share a combine and the income for each increases, then eventually they will be rich enough to afford, say, two groups of five, each sharing one combine. If disposable income keeps increasing, each farmer will end up having his own combine and we will thus have reached a complete privatization in consumption regarding this good. It can be shown (cf. Lindenberg, 1986) that a similar mechanism holds for positive externalities based on joint production rather than cost sharing (as is often found in families).

Once privatization in consumption for a particular good is complete, there will be no more sharing (regarding this good) and thus also no more norms with respect to sharing. But even if the privatization is not complete, the fact that sharing groups become smaller means that the veto principle will become less and less important. Norms will therefore be increasingly undermined by ad hoc situational agreements. Remember that this change does not just affect a particular norm but the whole norm hierachy including the importance of common values (and the importance of rituals for their dramatization). Socialization in the family will be strongly affected in the sense that the pressure from outside the home for norm conformity and shared-value-generating rituals decreases, and inside the home the pressure for maintaining the norm hierarchy also decreases because as fewer goods are being shared there are fewer negative externalities. Creating more privacy for every family member eventually leads to a situation in which everybody has his or her own room, entertainment electronics, telephone and bathroom. As a result, the family members will not have to work out concrete arrangements of sharing, nor do they have to pay much attention to higher order norms. Their interaction frequency will also decline. As a result they leave each other alone, do not try to judge the other's behaviour, and treat each other civilly but without much mutual involvement.

If norms weaken or even vanish, their by-product will also be affected: *less endowment with behavioural confirmation and positive affect*. The less behaviour is regulated by norms, the less it can be rewarded for conforming to the norms. This also holds for the possibility of the individual to be self-congratulatory about her own behaviour in anticipation of behavioural confirmation from others. As I have tried to show elsewhere (Lindenberg, 1986), there is little the family can do to create norms artificially once they realize that they are missing the by-products of social norms. Space does not permit me to repeat the argument here. Suffice it to say that norms will only develop where people cannot exit easily when norm conformity becomes a burden. Given the fact that little is still being shared in the family, it is impossible to create artifical exit barriers.

3.7.6. Norms and paid work

The same line of argument used above can be applied to paid work, and it makes clear why norms can still exist in the context of paid work even when they greatly decline in importance in home and in community life. Paid work is part of a joint production process (including the production of goods and services) with division of labour and thus with positive and negative externalities of the behaviour of one person for some or all of the other persons involved. This division is comparable to the sharing agreement discussed above and it will drive in a similar fashion the production of a hierarchy of norms. There are, however, considerable differences. First of all, the positive and negative externalities may not necessarily apply to the people you work with. Instead, they may affect supervisors, bosses, people in other departments, clients and other individuals removed from direct interaction. This may prevent the production or mobilization of higher order norms by the interacting indivi- duals, in which case these higher order norms and the sanctioning system will be *imposed on* rather than *created by* the interacting individuals. Also, shared values will not be easily dramatized and transaction costs will be manipulated by incentive schemes. In such circumstances, there are norms and sactions, but there are few positive externalities and thus not much behavioural confirmation is to be expected as a by-product of doing your work (cf. Coleman, 1990). The second important difference with the home is that children ordinarily are not socialized in the context of paid work. Thus the world of paid work will have to deal with adults that have been socialized in a certain way. If norms played only a small role during childhood socialization, it will be more difficult to make people comply to norms in the work place.

Yet, work organization will have to deal with the production of behavioural confirmation and thus with the creation of a work organization that resembles a larger sharing group with strong positive externalities. The reason for that can be gleaned from the arguments presented so far. We argued above that the home and the community at large become less efficient contexts for the production of endowment with behavioural confirmation. Since the context of paid work does produce norms it is in that respect able in principle to be an alternative to home and community (which would be especially important for women and for men in low status positions). A third possibility is the context of recreation, especially sports. Yet, since paid work also offers occupational status and income, it likely that this context will be the most important alternative to home and community. As a consequence, *there will be an increasing pressure (especially from married women of richer households and from lower status men) on work organizations to provide an efficient context for the endowment with behavioural confirmation.* This implies that the work organization would have to adapt in such a way that the norm hierarchy described for sharing groups can develop for the interacting groups in the organization. This may also imply a restructuring of tasks, of authority relations, of monitoring (sanctioning) arrangements, and of incentive schemes (cf. Lindenberg, 1988). To the degree that work organizations adapt their governance structures in this direction, the attractiveness of entering the labour force for women will increase and the relative importance of children for the production of social approval will decrease even more.

3.7.7. The status of life style

As the general level of welfare increases through increasing disposable income (and public goods privisions via the state), the life styles that are a by-product of making a home become generally more similar, and special efforts have to be made to still reap status from life styles (cf. Hirsch, 1978). In addition, with social norms on the decline, there will be less social control of life style and thus also less behavioural confirmation for the "right" life style. Even fashion is decreasing its grip in this respect. Quite generally, as it becomes less socially rewarding, life style is likely to shift more from the social approval production function to the physical well-being production function, possibly (but not likely) conflicting with "home."

3.8. Conclusion

In this paper, an attempt was made to introduce some traditional sociological insights, especially about the importance of social approval, into the discussion of fertility and female labour market behaviour in such a way, that the translation to the economic model building approach would be possible and maybe even inviting. The paper attempted to draw particular attention to the following issues:

a.   the importance of a constraint-driven heuristics, with general human goals and social production functions as means for reaching these goals;
b.   the pervasive influence of the fundamental exchange on social production functions and the gender division of labour;
c.   the workings of different forms of social approval with regard to family and labour market;
d.   the dynamic elements behind a slow but thorough sea change in fertility and labour market behaviour of women: the privatization of consumption.

With the last point, it hopes to make a particular contribution to the economic approach, by pointing to the great limitation of looking at or worrying about cross-sectional income effects. This line of reasoning should also be relevant for the inclusion of changes in governance structures of work organizations in the analysis of fertility and labour market behaviour. Work organization will have to attract an increasing part of the labour force by offering the opportunity for behavioural confirmation. If governance structures adapt to provide just that, they in turn will increase female labour market participation and lower fertility.

Part II
Preferences

DE GUSTIBUS CONFUSI SUMUS ?

Thomas K. Burch
Department of Sociology
Faculty of Social Science
The University of Western Ontario
LONDON, Ontario N6A 5C2
Canada

4.1. Introduction

The central point of this note is that a variety of terms, including *tastes* and *preferences*, continue to be used indiscriminately to refer to a number of conceptually and empirically distinct realities, some of which are properties of an individual actor (subjective states of respondents), some of which are properties of social systems. These states are conceptually distinct in the sense that many theories of behaviour as well as everyday experience suggest that they are different - what I want to do, what society says I should do, what I feel I must do and what I intend to do are not necessarily and not always the same. They also are empirically distinct in the sense that their measures may show relatively little covariance and seem to represent different underlying dimensions.

Illustrations of the conceptual problem are taken from literature on tastes generally and specifically on their role in the study of fertility and work.

Empirical illustrations are provided by data from the 1984 Canadian Fertility Survey, which asked a number of questions relating to subjective states of women of childbearing age (N = 5,315) with respect to relationships, children, work and personal freedom.

A methodological conclusion is that future surveys, whether cross-sectional or longitudinal, might devote more effort to the measurement of these confounded concepts (or dimensions).

4.2. Background

A classic reference on this topic is the article by Stigler and Becker (1977) entitled "De gustibus non est disputandum." In this influential paper, how did

Stigler and Becker define *tastes* ? The simple answer is that they didn't; that is, the article does not provide a formal substantive definition of the term. It is likely that they took for granted the standard definition in economics, namely anything pertaining to an actor or his/her choice behaviour that cannot be subsumed under the concepts of *prices* and *income*. For Stigler and Becker, as for economists generally, *tastes* is a residual concept.

This residual character of tastes in behavioural theory was pointed out as long ago as 1937 by Talcott Parsons in *The Structure of Social Action*, which devotes a full four and one-half pages to a section entitled "Residual Categories" (1937, I, pp. 16-20). Using a metaphor of light and darkness, Parsons comments: "Every (scientific) system, including both its theoretical propositions and its main empirical insights, may be visualized as an illuminated spot enveloped by darkness. The logical name for the darkness is, in general, 'residual categories' " (p. 17). He goes on to note that " . . . one kind of theoretical work consists precisely in the carving out from residual categories of definite positively defined concepts and their verification in empirical investigation" (p. 18).

For Becker and Stigler, as for most economists, tastes and preferences remain at least in shadow if not darkness. But what sorts of things do they include under *tastes* ? A close reading of their article yields the following list of "things" that are more or less identified with *tastes*: desires; interests; sentiments; feelings; "modes of thinking and acting which prevail throughout the community" (quoting J.S. Mill); habits; maxims; traditions; values. A similar list could easily be compiled from other sources in the economics literature. (For a broader review of the variety of ideational or subjective elements invoked to explain behaviour, see Burch, 1987).

Turning to the literature on fertility, it is worth citing Easterlin's identification of *tastes* with *norms*: " . . . the principal emphasis of sociology is on the tendency of behavior to conform to 'social norms,' the conceptual embodiment of preferences" (Easterlin, 1969, p. 133), and Ryder's eloquent rejection of such an identification:

> "Norms are not just another discipline's jargon for tastes and preferences. The distinction is crucial between them. . . . When tastes and preferences are employed for some purpose more elevating than circular reasoning, they promote research into the properties of individuals, whereas norms are properties of organized groups. " (Ryder, 1973).

A useful but neglected formalization of Ryder's point is provided by Fishbein (1972), who conceptualizes attitudes (defined as readiness to act in a certain way toward a certain object) as functions of an individual inclination and of normative influences outside the individual.

The conceptualization of norms as being outside of and transcending the individual is a key idea in the Durkheimian tradition of social theory (norms are characterized by "exteriority and constraint"), and still finds expression in contemporary thinking. Namboodiri, for example, in a critique of Beckerian microeconomics and its notion that norms will be violated if the rewards are great enough and the price is right (1980), comments: "Many sociologists ... would argue that in practice adherence to norms is non-negotiable, and, hence, immune to economic bribe. Norms are there to be adhered to, no matter what the perceived price tag is." (Note: The validity of such an assertion presumably depends on one's definition and classification of *norms*, and, depending on definition, it may apply to some norms but not others.)

The literature on female labour-force participation and fertility provides similar illustrations. Cramer (1980), for example, generally neglects tastes in trying to untangle the relationships between work and fertility, but clearly equates them with: plans; intentions; expectations; attitudes; goals. He does distinguish "social norms and individual fertility preferences" (p. 187) but only in passing.

Even the best literature on the fertility-work nexus does not seem to have escaped the problem. Bagozzi and Van Loo (1982), for example, proxy taste for work by an item dealing with a woman's *perception* as to the extent that the burden associated with housework *would* be shared with her husband *if* she were employed, and by another item on the wife's *felt obligation* to work to meet family needs. On the face of it, the former would seem to be an expectation or a hope, the latter a subjective normative factor; neither seems to be a *preference* in the sense of a wish or desire for one thing relative to another. Bagozzi and Van Loo also extend the concept of *tastes* to include unconscious as well as conscious feelings, an interesting but arguable innovation - the argument would be not about attention to un- or sub-conscious factors but to their equation with *tastes* and to their measurement (in the case at hand, by church attendance).

It is well understood, of course, that Bagozzi and Van Loo, like the rest of us, must often make do with interview items that are available, items that are not specifically designed to measure concepts that our theories or models might require. A particularly sticky problem in the case at hand is the difficulty (some would say "impossibility") of measuring social norms from individual survey data. The most one can get is some idea of respondent consensus on what they *perceive* as the relevant social norms in a particular realm of behaviour.

4.3. Canadian Fertility Survey data

It is easy to spin out conceptual distinctions, and contrary to the canon of parsimony in science to go farther in this direction than is necessary or fruitful for explanation. Empirical work sometimes demonstrates that a particular conceptual elaboration collapses onto one underlying dimension, or adds nothing to explained variance. Falbo and Becker, for example, have shown that at least in one case, Fishbein's value times expectancy model was too elaborate; salient values alone provided as much predictive power as did the combination of values with an expectancy measure (Falbo and Becker, 1980).

As a contribution to the empirical examination of these issues, this note examines the content and co-variation of twenty or so different interview items contained in the 1984 Canadian Fertility Survey (Population Studies Centre, UWO, 1984). The items, varying in wording and format, all deal in one way or another with the woman's subjective states vis-à-vis children, work, or their interrelationships. Included are items dealing with perceived norms, but as noted above, it remains an open question whether these can be interpeted as measures of the norms themselves. Table 1 describes each item and gives marginals in percents. Each item has been assigned a code (A1, B2, etc.) for easier reference in what follows.

Items A1 through A5, whether by accident or design, appear to refer to *tastes* in the classic economic sense (see Becker, 1976, p. 137), and refer to what the respondent thinks is important to *her* happiness. (Note: Some economists would disagree, arguing that a preference for A can only be measured, if at all, with specific reference to other goods B, C, D, etc.).

B1 and B4 are similar, but the wording does not contain such a clear reference to personal happiness or desires; one could, for instance, agree that a child provides a goal in life that nothing else can, but still not strongly desire a child for oneself. B2 and B3 refer to perceived disadvantages of a child or children; the latter item is fairly obvious, and 94 percent of respondents agreed with it. Item C relates to the perception of conflicts between having children and working outside the home, in particular limits children impose on working. To some extent these items are tapping the respondent's perception of how having children affects people's lives generally.

Item D asks about the respondent's personal opinion as to the propriety of outside employment by women with young children. Items E1 and E2 ask about the woman's perception of what the "majority" of men find acceptable in the matter of employment outside the home, contingent on having or not having children. These items generally relate to perceived norms or role expectations.

Item F would seem to be tapping the woman's personal preferences for daycare arrangement. Item G asks about the motivation of "parents" (presumably parents in general) for having a second child, specifically, whether they are child-centered or parent-centered.

H1 through H3 ask about the respondent's personal opinion on the acceptability of divorce in the presence or absence of children. Item I relates to the acceptability of cohabitation by a divorced woman with children.

Clearly, these items cover a wide range of different subjective states - preferences, norms, perceptions -, as well as a wide range of behavioural referents - value of children, disadvantages of children, divorce, cohabitation, work, freedom, etc. What are the empirical relationships among them ?

An examination of the correlation matrix among these variables shows relatively few high or significant associations. A factor analysis (using SPSS-X varimax rotation procedures) of eighteen of the items relating to children, work, or child/work interrelations yields seven separate factors (see table 2). Most of the factors are readily interpreted in terms of the specific items with heavy loadings. Factor 2, for example, relates to *tastes* for family life; factor 5, to perceived male attitudes about female employment; factor 6, to disadvantages of children, and so forth.

Slightly different results are obtained depending on how specific items are coded, and when items are added or deleted (e.g., on intention to work until 60). But in every case, several factors emerge. Conceptual distinctions discussed above seem to have some basis also in empirical measurement.

Table 1. Frequency distributions on tastes and other subjective items.

(A) In order for you to be generally happy in life, is it very important, important, not very important or not at all important ...

	Very important	Important	Not very important	Not at all important
	(%)			
1) to have a lasting relationship as a couple	66	29	5	1
2) to be married	41	29	22	9
3) to have at least one child	40	31	20	8
4) to be able to take a job outside the home	32	40	21	7
5) to be free to do as you wish	43	45	11	2

(B) On the whole, would you say that you strongly agree, agree, disagree, or strongly disagree with the following statements ...

	Strongly agree	Agree	Disagree	Strongly disagree
	(%)			
1) having a child provides a goal in life that nothing else can	32	40	22	6
2) having children tends to distance the spouses from one another	2	16	50	32
3) becoming parents means taking on heavy responsibilities	56	38	5	2
4) having a child provides an irreplaceable source of affection	39	46	14	2

Table 1 (continued)

(C) For a woman, do you think that having young children reduces their work opportunities outside the home a lot, a fair amoung, not very much, or not at all ?

	A lot	Fair amount	Not very much	Not at all
	(%)			
	24	39	24	13

(D) In your opinion, is it acceptable for a woman who has a child *under three* to work outside the home ?

		(%)		
	Yes	73	No	27

(E) In general, do you believe that the majority of men accept fairly well that their wife (partner) work outside the home ?

		(%)		
1) when she has children	Yes	73	No	27
2) when she has no children	Yes	97	No	3

(F) When a woman who has a child under three decides to work outside the home, which one of the following three childcare solutions *is the best* ?

	(%)
a babysitter at home	63
taking the child to a babysitter's home	7
a daycare center	29
multiple response	1

Table 1 (continued)

(G) In your opinion, do parents have a second child in order to create
a better environment for the children *or rather* for their own personal
satisfaction ?

	(%)
better environment for children	50
parent's satisfaction	40
both	10

(H) Do you approve without reservation, approve with reservations,
or completely disapprove of divorce in the following circumstances ?

	No reservations	Reservations	Disapprove
	(%)		
1) the couple have very young children	17	55	28
2) the couple have teenagers	28	55	17
3) the couple have no children	65	28	7

(I) Do you find it acceptable for a divorced woman to live with her children
and a new partner without being married to him ?

	(%)
Yes	54
No	46

Table 2. Factor analysis of eighteen interview items on subjective
   perceptions concerning children and work: rotated factor matrix.

				Factors			
Item	#1	#2	#3	#4	#5	#6	#7
A1	.02	*.59*	.08	-.03	.06	-.07	.03
A2	-.15	*.78*	.04	-.03	.03	.03	.00
A3	-.10	*.63*	.33	.09	-.02	.09	.00
A4	.03	.04	-.12	*.73*	-.07	.14	-.07
A5	.06	-.02	.02	*.64*	.05	-.21	.29
B1	-.10	.21	*.74*	-.04	.00	.06	.03
B2	.07	-.02	.02	.03	-.20	*.62*	-.01
B3	-.03	-.04	.04	.02	.20	*.73*	.15
B4	-.03	.03	*.80*	-.06	.00	.01	-.03
C	.02	-.02	-.02	.03	-.04	.16	*.82*
D	.15	-.14	.00	*.51*	.20	.17	-.37
E1	.02	.01	.05	.08	*.70*	.06	-.28
E2	.02	.05	-.05	-.03	*.75*	-.10	.16
G	-.02	.27	-.08	-.03	-.15	.22	-.19
H1	*.83*	-.11	-.11	.03	.06	.02	-.04
H2	*.89*	-.09	-.10	.06	.03	.05	-.01
H3	*.74*	-.01	.01	.06	-.03	.01	.05
I	*.35*	-.38	.22	.28	-.03	.15	-.02

Notes:
High loadings (0.5 or better) are in italic type.
The eighteen items had various response options (approve/disapprove, yes/no,
acceptable/unacceptable, etc.). These were recoded so that 1 represented a
positive response, 0 a neutral response (incl. don't know), and -1 a negative
response. Alternate codings (e.g., dummy, original arbitrary scale without
collapsing) produce very similar overall results.

The general pattern observed in table 2 is also obtained when separate analyses are made for women under thirty and those thirty and over. There are differences in detail, as might be expected after almost two decades of revolutionary change in family life and the role of women. But the similarities are greater than the differences.

The picture is not entirely a tidy one. Factor 4, for example, "mixes" two taste items with one relating to the respondent's normative judgements. That is, the procedure associates empirically items one might wish to hold distinct conceptually.

It is interesting that tastes for work and tastes for freedom end up in the same factor. One suspects that a different result would be obtained for male respondents, but for women, presumably, work represents freedom from traditional domestic roles.

4.4. Discussion

The above results suggest that more than one or two items might be needed to map the subjective landscape in a way that will lead to an understanding of the work/fertility relationship (as well as demographic behaviour generally). There are several different dimensions - tastes, perceptions of reality, expectations, perceived norms - in any one content area, and there are several different content areas - work, children, daycare, leisure, intimate relationships.

The key question, of course, is whether this elaboration of the subjective realm leads to better models of fertility, work, and their mutual relationships. Preliminary work along these lines on the Canadian Fertility Survey shows: a) moderate associations of tastes for work and for children with education and frequency of church attendance (tables 3 and 4); b) interactions among taste and behavioural items relating to work and children and perception of conflict between work and children, and interactions among work, taste for work and fertility. The latter findings emerge in loglinear analyses studying interrelationships with no particular causal assumptions.

Such analysis is greatly hampered by the cross-sectional design of the survey, with "attitudinal" items measured at time of interview. But the richness of the subjective items and the above results seem to warrant further work.

Table 3. Tastes for children and work by educational level.

	Years of Education		
	0-8	9-12	13+
	(%)		
Importance of having at least one child:			
Very important	55	43	36
Important	33	31	31
Not very important	8	19	23
Not at all important	4	7	10

> Somer's D (symmetric) = 0.11
> Contingency coeff.   = 0.14
> Cramer's V   = 0.10

	Years of Education		
	0-8	9-12	13+
	(%)		
Importance of taking job outside the home:			
Very important	24	26	39
Important	35	42	39
Not very important	27	25	16
Not at all important	14	8	5

> Somer's D (symmetric) = 0.16
> Contingency coeff.   = 0.18
> Cramer's V   = 0.13

Thomas K. Burch

Table 4. Tastes for children and work by frequency of church attendance.

	Frequency of church attendance				
	Weekly	Monthly	Few times /year	Rarely	Never
	(%)				
Importance of having at least one child:					
Very important	51	47	39	34	28
Important	29	33	34	33	27
Not very important	16	16	20	21	29
Not at all important	4	4	6	12	17

Somer's D (symmetric) = 0.17
Contingency coeff.   = 0.22
Cramer's V   = 0.13

	Frequency of church attendance				
	Weekly	Monthly	Few times /year	Rarely	Never
	(%)				
Importance of taking job outside the home:					
Very important	24	28	33	37	38
Important	37	44	44	41	42
Not very important	28	22	20	17	15
Not at all important	11	5	6	5	5

Somer's D (symmetric) = -0.13
Contingency coeff.   = 0.17
Cramer's V   = 0.10

Current comment on research design often emphasizes the need for longitudinal or prospective designs to measure tastes prior to and therefore presumably independent of behaviours they might affect. The results presented here suggest also more attention to interview schedules and procedures (e.g., probes) that would distinguish what seem to be distinct subjective realities.

In this connection, it appears that the specific wording of items A1 through A5 provides a good start towards measurement of tastes in the classic sense of that term - how important the respondent thinks various things are for *her own* happiness.

SHORTCUTS AS PITFALLS ?
WAYS OF MEASURING CHILDBEARING PREFERENCES AND INTENTIONS

Freddy Deven and Sabien Bauwens
Centrum voor Bevolkings- en Gezinsstudiën
Markiesstraat 1
1000 BRUSSELS
Belgium

5.1. Introduction

Measuring childbearing preferences and intentions, although commonly practised, is considered to be a strenuous exercise. In Flanders (Belgium), the first large-scale fertility survey was launched in 1966. Since then, this kind of effort was repeated periodically. Accordingly, there is room for a comparative reflection in retrospect.

This paper more specifically considers our involvement in the 3rd and 4th fertility survey, the "Survey on Family Development" (= NEGO) in Flanders, Belgium. Common to both empirical endeavours is the a priori of a large-scale survey, the use of a structured questionnaire and a sample of three to five thousand respondents.

First, the type and rationale of our data collection will be considered in retrospect. We aim to critically look at the possibilities and limitations of our measurement tools. The analysis will consider specifically the measurement of family size preferences, the impact of significant others, and the (predictive value of) childbearing intentions.

Viewed against the background of the increasingly sophisticated models being developed to study reproductive behaviour, the drawbacks can be considered to which extent a piecemeal measurement of the central concepts of the models brings about incomplete and/or biased knowledge. Do our "shortcuts" necessarily lead to pitfalls ?

5.2. Background

Since shortly after its creation, one of the main projects of the Population and Family Study Centre (CBGS) has been one of a broad data collection on the fertility and fertility regulating behaviour of the female population in

Belgium. In 1966, a first large-scale survey included a representative sample of married women below forty-one. The second survey (1971) involved women aged 30-34 years.

For the 3rd "Survey on Family Development" (=NEGO 3, 1975-1976) a major part on motivational issues related to reproductive behaviour was included. The overall aim of the NEGO-3 survey remained to provide basic data on the fertility and fertility regulating behaviour of women. This time, the representative, stratified sample included 20-45 year old women as well as married women of the age cohort 15-19 (all respondents, n = 4,700). A subgroup of couples (n = 700) was also included.

5.3. A value-of-children module

The development of a "value-of-children" (VOC) subset of questions within the 3rd "Survey on Family Development" predominantly relied on (1) the preliminary research of Fawcett and Arnold (1973) in Hawaii on the value of children to parents; (2) exploratory work in a clinical setting; and (3) the results of the NEGO-3 pilot survey combined with those of a similar initiative in the Netherlands (Niphuis-Nell and Moors, 1979).

The VOC-module consisted of a semi-structured questionnaire for personal interviews at home. It included open-ended questions on the advantages and disadvantages of parenthood versus childlessness, as well as on the perceived reasons for the declining birth rate in the country. Besides the conventional single questions, childbearing preferences were tapped more extensively through a simplified version of the Family Size Utility Function (Terhune and Kaufman, 1973; Debusschere and Deven, 1981). Finally, a list of Likert-type items measuring beliefs related to the value of children to parents and two structured sets of "positive" and "negative" parenthood items (importance ratings) were included (Deven, 1979, 1982). Due to time constraints, only one of the sets of items mentioned above could be submitted, dependent on the childbearing intention of each respondent below 35 years old.

5.3.1. NEGO-3 findings

From the overall findings, especially those from the subsample of couples are looked at.

Considering their childbearing preferences and intentions, a parity-specific analysis showed that at most 59% of the couples perceived each other's preferred family size correctly. It was lowest among one-child parents. On average, about one fourth of the couples showed no concordance at all. Finally, in case of a partial concordance more women than men seemed to perceive correctly the partner's preferred number of children (Deven, 1983).

Table 1 presents the childbearing intention of couples of which the woman is 25-29 years old. This information was collected by a dichotomous question. Obviously, the intention to have another child sharply decreases with the actual number of children. More interestingly, one can notice the discrepancy of the childbearing intention among a number of couples. For example, almost one fifth of the couples having two children hold conflicting intentions related to future childbearing.

Through another study involving a third of the respondents from the NEGO-3 survey, a number of follow-up data enabled us to check among others the predictive value of the childbearing intention. Couples intending to have a/another child at time one (1975-1976) had on average 0.90 children, those considering their childbearing career as closed had 1.69 children.

Setting additional eligibility requirements in accordance with the work of Westoff and Ryder (1977), 195 female respondents were left for comparison from the subsample of couples. At the individual level, 54% of women intending to have a/another child was as yet inconsistent at time two (three years later) compared to 9% of women intending not to have a/another child in the future. The effect of the actual number of children at time one is substantial (Deven, 1983).

A simplified version of the Family Size Utility Function (= FSUF, Terhune and Kaufman, 1973) was included to counteract the shortcomings of the single-question measurement of family size preference. Our work documents that a coherent set of measures can be obtained with this simplified FSUF on the condition that the basic data from which they are derived are of good quality (Debusschere and Deven, 1981). It especially provides useful information on the attitude towards "extreme" family sizes (< 1, ≥ 4) of respondents entering their reproductive career.

Considering 25-29 year old women and their partner, a substantial amount of similarity is found in their expected amount of (dis)satisfaction with different family sizes. Controlling for parity, this similarity decreases with their actual number of children.

Table 1. The childbearing intention of couples, by their actual family size.
NEGO 3, 25-29 year old women and their partner.

Childbearing intention	Actual family size *			
	0	1	2	3
Yes, both	80	49	11	13
Yes, woman only	6	10	13	8
Yes, man only	4	5	6	3
No, both	11	33	67	75
Incomplete data	-	3	3	0
n = 100%	138	263	221	61

* Data for couples with actual family size ≥ 4 are not shown (n = 19).

Much effort went into documenting the perceptions of women and men in Flanders, particularly towards the anticipated benefits and costs of parenthood in general and a number of family sizes in particular. Among a large set of parenthood items a few are clearly emphasized differently by women and men. Looking at the most important expectancies among childless couples in Flanders (1975-1976), men expect more strongly that a child will strengthen the relationship and provide them a goal to work and live for. Expectant mothers stress more the pleasures to be derived from interacting with the child. Mothers of one child expect significantly more than their partner that a sibling will be beneficial to their first child. Among those couples not intending to have another child, women systematically expect a greater burden as well as more impediments on their labour force participation compared to their partner. Fathers do express more concern about possible complications during pregnancy and/or delivery, about the financial burden as well as about their partner's unwillingness to have another child (Deven, 1979, 1982).

5.3.2. In retrospect

It is considered that much of these data concern the perceptions of the respondents, particularly towards their anticipated satisfactions and costs of parenthood. Although the limits of this methodology are clear, it was felt that a broad and subjectively meaningful set of data was obtained (e.g. Busfield and Paddon, 1977).

Especially during the second half of the seventies the results of similar and other kind of research efforts became available. Our findings on the values and disvalues of children to parents revealed similar to comparable data from large-scale surveys in other industrialized countries such as the Netherlands and the USA (Bulatao, 1979). More generally, Bulatao (1981) comprehensively documents a number of components involved in the childbearing decision-making process, emphasizing as well the importance of a parity-specific analysis.

Besides the "value of children" approach other social-psychological approaches were explored as well. Applying the "Fishbein-model" to the domain of contraceptive use and childbearing intentions revealed successful (e.g. Werner *et al.*, 1975), also within the context of short-term longitudinal studies (Vinokur-Kaplan, 1978; Davidson and Jaccard, 1979). Such a subjective expected utility approach, also used by Townes *et al.* (1980), implies a nuanced set of questions in order to predict the childbearing intention.

The work of Beckman (1979) is based on the social exchange theory. She too opted for a "shortcut measurement" by utilizing importance ratings of the perceived benefits and costs of (additional) childbearing. The argument is that a salience or importance rating may already include a person's internal assessment of likelihood as well as an affective component. An outstanding example of a shortcut as pitfall ?

Bagozzi and Van Loo (1978b) made a strong case within their social-psychological model to take the husband-and-wife relationship as the unit of analysis. Evidence accumulated that two-sex regression models predict fertility (intention) better than wife-only models do (e.g. Fried *et al.*, 1980). The volume of Burch (1980) clearly documents a variety of possible perspectives related to the study of human reproductive behaviour.

5.4. NEGO 4: improving the fertility-related measurement

The design of another large-scale fertility survey came about in the early 1980s. For the section "parenthood" of the NEGO-4 survey a number of considerations guided the work. Comparability with the previous survey was an overall aim of the NEGO-4 project. A representative sample of 20-44 year old women (n=3,100) provided the respondents for this research. Budgetary constraints made it impossible for us to include again a (sub)sample of couples.

5.4.1. Additional measurement tools

Our experience with the VOC-module in the previous survey (1975-1976) gave way to a number of modifications. Those components being given more specific attention in the NEGO-4 survey are briefly discussed below.

First, results from the previous survey document specific birth interval patterns. Do young, childless women also share preferences or beliefs related to an ideal timing, say between marriage and the birth of a first child or an appropriate age (for women and men) to stop childbearing ? Single questions have been submitted to trigger information about the existence of a "parenthood mandate", "proper" reproductive age limits (if any) for women and men as well as about the time interval considered ideal between parity 0-1 and 1-2.

Second, especially the response patterns to the parenthood items show the importance attributed to her partner and child/ren, if any. Previous research indicates that most social pressure concerning reproduction is expected and received from close relatives, especially for non-parents (e.g. Ory, 1978; Clay and Zuiches, 1980). This issue is felt particularly difficult to grasp as most respondents deny that the reaction of those people will have any influence on their reproductive decision-making (e.g. Fried and Udry, 1980). We therefore attempted to measure the possible impact of some "significant others" in a multimethod way (see below).

Third, the set of parenthood items was reconsidered in the light of the experience with our previous research. Missing components such as the evaluation of the experience with a first/second child or the possible impact on one's health were included.

Fourth, it is recognized that reproductive outcome only presents a final stage in a process of events (e.g. Hass, 1974). Miller (1980; 1986) for example documents the importance of instrumental behaviour (proception) between the intention (becoming pregnant) and a reproductive event (conception).

A number of variables were added to measure the perceived behavioural control over becoming pregnant and having or not having a/another child. For example, we inquired about the probability of having a/another child in the near future and about the woman's perceived fecundity and reproductive health. Besides a detailed set of questions about past and present contraceptive use,

women were also asked to evaluate the effectiveness of their contraceptive
method as well as to express their behavioural intention if an unwanted pregnancy were to occur.

Finally, the woman's childbearing intention as well as her perception of
that of her partner was elaborated into a five-code variable, leaving room for
the expression of uncertainty and ambivalence.

The major findings on these variables are presented below.

5.4.2. NEGO-4 findings

Table 2 clearly shows the strong relationship between the type of childbearing
intention and the woman's parity status. Noticable remains the amount of
ambivalence and uncertainly expressed by 20-34 year old women at different
parity levels.

Respondents were also asked to evaluate their actual number of children
by comparing it with their preferred family size (table 3). Did they consider
it was equal, higher or lower ? To what extent does it coincide with their
childbearing intention ? In general, among women who consider that their actual
family size equals or exceeds their preferred one a small minority still
intends to have another child. On the other hand, among women who have at
present fewer children than they would prefer, a significant minority does not
intend to have a/another child.

For 20-34 year old women in the early 1980s three expectancies are most
strongly linked with their intention not to have a/another child. A too
uncertain and gloomy future ranks highest, especially among the lower educated
women. Next comes the possible impediment on their labour force participation.
Higher educated women significantly more expect this, being more professionally
involved and sharing more equally household tasks with their partner. Finally,
the partner's unwillingness is also strongly stressed by (the lowest educated)
housewives and unemployed women (Bauwens and Deven, 1989).

Positive parenthood expectancies most strongly held relate predominantly
to the affective dimension (e.g. the pleasure of having a/another child around)
and to familism (e.g. a family needs children). Considering a sibling to be
very important for their first child is clearly found among those intending
to have a second child. Contrary to our data from the mid seventies, the
expectancy that a child cements the couple is not held as strongly.

Table 2. Childbearing intentions, by their actual family size.
         NEGO 4, 20-34 year old women

| Childbearing | Actual family size | | | | |
intention	0	1	2	3+	total
No!	11	37	65	80	39.2
No, unless	4	6	8	6	5.8
I still doubt	11	13	12	10	11.8
Yes, unless	6	4	3	1	4.3
Yes!	67	40	12	3	38.9
n = 100%	706	522	529	173	1930

Table 3. Childbearing intentions, by an evaluation of the preferred
         and actual family size. NEGO 4, 20-34 year old women.

| Childbearing | Actual versus preferred family size | | |
intention	Act.< Pref.	Act.= Pref.	Act.> Pref.
No!	13	81	92
Doubt	23	17	4
Yes!	64	2	4
n = 100%	1176	670	75

Table 4 shows a way of looking at the possible impact of normative pressures
stemming from (some) significant others on the women's childbearing intention.
Women were asked whether they experienced that having a/another child or not
having one was important or not for the partner, the parents or the child(ren),
if any.

Overall, the way women perceive that (not) having a/another child matters,
especially for their partner, significantly influences their childbearing
intention. For those evaluating their actual number of children below their
preferred one, a substantial difference shows both for the partner and the
parents. For women whose actual family size equals their preferred one the

partner's impact becomes less explicit whereas the possible impact from the parents almost disappears.

Using stepwise regression analysis, 49% of variance of the childbearing intention of 20-34 year old women is covered (data not shown). Among the set of variables included (see table 5), the majority is of a social-demographic nature. A few social-psychological variables are included as well: the possible normative pressure from the partner and the parents, the amount to which a "parenthood mandate" is held (e.g. the strongly held belief that a couple ultimately should have children), the family size considered ideal at present in Flanders and a three-code variable expressing a "traditional", "mixed" or "emancipated" division of household tasks. Finally, two social-biological variables are added, the woman's perception of her fecundity and her reproductive health.

Table 4. Childbearing pressure from partner and/or parents related to the woman's childbearing intention, by her evaluated family size. NEGO 4, 20-34 years old women.

Childbearing intention woman	Childbearing pressure from			
	Partner		Parents	
	C+	C-	C+	C-
A. Actual family size < Preferred family size				
No!	5	32	6	24
doubt	11	45	14	42
yes!	84	23	80	34
n=100%	306	128	248	71
B. Actual family size = Preferred family size				
No!	70	90	74	80
doubt	27	9	26	20
Yes!	3	1	0	0
n=100%	73	197	50	81
C. Actual family size > Preferred family size				
data not shown (n < 26)				

Note:
C+ = important to have a/another child;
C- = important *not* to have a/another child in the family.

Table 5. Stepwise regression analysis of childbearing intention, by actual family size. NEGO 4, 20-34 year old women.

	actual family size=0		actual family size=1		actual family size=2	
	R^2	B	R^2	B	R^2	B
R^2	42.3%		43.7%		21.4%	
Intercept		2.55		0.94		1.43
Age 1)	7.4	-0.57	18.4	-0.71	9.0	-0.50
Educational level 2)	3.8	+0.22	14.8	+0.58	1.8	+0.19
Religious affiliation 3)	1.2	-0.11	n.s.	n.s.	n.s.	n.s.
Family income 4)	n.s.	n.s.	n.s.	n.s.	n.s.	n.s.
Woman's income 5)	n.s.	n.s.	n.s.	n.s.	0.9	+0.06
Employment D1 6)	6.1	-0.40	0.9	-0.49	n.s.	n.s.
Employment D2 7)	n.s.	n.s.	n.s.	n.s.	n.s.	n.s.
Housing	n.s.	n.s.	n.s.	n.s.	n.s.	n.s.
NP/partner 8)	24.1	+0.90	6.7	+0.56	5.6	+0.49
NP/parents 8)	n.s.	n.s.	0.4	+0.23	0.8	-0.29
Parenthood mandate	4.0	+0.23	n.s.	n.s.	0.8	+0.13
Ideal family size	n.s.	n.s.	0.9	n.s.	n.s.	n.s.
Division household tasks 9)	0.6	-0.60	n.s.	n.s.	1.1	+1.14
Fecundity	n.s.	n.s.	n.s.	n.s.	1.4	+0.29
Reproductive health	0.8	+0.46	1.4	+0.44	n.s.	n.s.

Notes:

The standard significance of 0.15 in stepwise regression analyses is set as the level of inclusion. Variables not meeting this criterion are excluded from the model. The total proportion of variance in childbearing intention explained by the set of included variables, is given by the R^2 above. Each variable that contributes significantly is characterized by two values: a partial R^2 indicating the relative weight in the total explained variance and an unstandardized B-parameter estimating the direction and magnitude of the relationship between the independent and the dependent variable.

n.s. = not significant

1) 20-24, 25-29, 30-34 years
2) Primary to university level (5 codes)
3) Catholic (3 codes), non-religious, Atheist
4) <35,000 Bfr, 35,000-60,000 Bfr, >60,000 Bfr (3 codes)
5) No income, <25,000 Bfr, >25,000 Bfr
6) Housewife full-time (dummy variable: no, yes)
7) Seeking employment (dummy variable: no, yes)
8) Normative pressure (2 codes : no/yes)
9) Amount of segregation (3 codes)

Parity-specific analyses for the same age group leave somewhat more of the variance unexplained (see table 5). For childless women, their age and educational level clearly contribute although most variance relates to the perceived importance the (further) childbearing holds for her partner (e.g. normative pressure of partner). The "parenthood mandate" contributes to some extent.

The childbearing intention of mothers of one child is influenced by their age and their educational level. The partner's option keeps some impact. For 20-34 year old women with two children this general set of variables is unable to shed much light on their further childbearing decision-making.

5.4. Discussion

Considering the overall theme of this book, the work of our colleagues analysing the patterns of labour force participation is summarized below.

Pauwels *et al.* (1987) document that within the overall rise in female labour market participation, the highest participation rates are noted for 20-34 year old women. Multiple classification analysis reveals that the educational level of Flemish women is the most important determinant for a continued participation in the labour market. Next comes their family size. Beyond a certain threshold, the partner's net income negatively influences their labour market involvement.

Impens (1987) notices that considerable less attention has been given so far to the impact of female unemployment on the timing and intensity of child-bearing. His multivariate proportional hazards analysis reveals a significant birth probability reducing impact of unemployment. This effect is parity-specific, direct as well as indirect. It declines however with an increased educational level, as far as the first birth is concerned. It implies that a hampered female labour market participation (i.e. unemployment) can have an even greater effect on childbearing than employment as such.

Analysing the data for 20-34 year old women from the NEGO-4 survey in fact provides a picture of the childbearing preferences, intentions and reproductive behaviour of most women of the babyboom generation in Flanders (Belgium). Surveys such as NEGO 4 involve three thousand respondents or more. It is felt this prerequisite severely conditions the type of data collection and measurement, bringing us to a number of concessions and shortcuts.

Using the simplified version of the Family Size Utility Function clearly restricts the possibility of interpretation. By not presenting the different family sizes for pairwise comparisons, the preferences are deducted by the researcher, not by the respondents themselves.

Collecting data from women only does not allow for the testing of any model in which information from both partners is a central assumption. Relying solely on the woman's perception of her partners' childbearing preferences and/or intention clearly puts the researcher at risk of measuring to some extent wishful thinking. Notwithstanding these limitations, we take it from the previous survey experience (NEGO 3) that women on average seem to provide more correctly this type of information needed about their partner than men do. Moreover, data about the way respondents perceive preferences from one or more significant others are deemed valuable in order to construct a normative pressure-component.

A substantial limitation remains the shortcut that the response pattern on the parenthood-items does not include all respondents. In 1982-1983, only those respondents expressing (some) uncertainty about their future childbearing were submitted both to "positive" and "negative" parenthood items. Accordingly, a key social-psychological variable had to be left out from the multivariate analysis.

Among scholars studying fertility (regulating) behaviour from a social-psychological perspective, the Fishbein model or the theory of reasoned action (Ajzen and Fishbein, 1980) became "popular". This subjective expected utility approach accumulated a fair amount of evidence in support, also through its application in the domain of childbearing and fertility regulation. At the same time, a number of shortcomings were pointed at and some fundamental problems remain unsolved (e.g. Falbo and Becker, 1980; Liska, 1984; Bagozzi, 1986; Burnkrant and Page, 1988). The concepts employed are basically motivational in nature. One crucial assumption in the model of Fishbein and Ajzen is that the behaviour has to be volitional. A complex behaviour such as human reproduction can hardly be defined as purely volitional. Among others, a modest set of social-biological variables in our research indicates that the conceptive, contraceptive and childbearing capacity of women and men clearly interfere. The final outcome certainly does not immediately follow the intention whereas the assumption of an additive, recursive causal structure seems inadequate.

The authors themselves tackled the requirement that the behaviour under consideration be under volitional control. Closer scrutiny indeed reveals that childbearing wishes and preferences are quite often subject to the influence of factors beyond one's control. Accordingly, Ajzen and Madden considered that

> "most intended behaviors are best considered goals whose attainment is subject to some degree of uncertainty. We can thus speak of behavior-goal units and of intentions as plans of action in pursuit of behavioral goals." (Ajzen and Madden, 1986, p. 456)

To remedy this problem Ajzen (1985) submitted a "theory of planned behavior". It extends the former model by including the concept of perceived behavioural control which bears similarities to the concept of locus of control as well as with that of self-efficacy beliefs.

Our attempts to study reproductive behaviour within the context of a large-scale survey certainly bear several implications for future research. Foremost, the explicit need to cast our set of variables into a coherent framework. The overall data collection represents a multidisciplinary approach in which the fertility and fertility regulating behaviour of the population is studied in various loosely integrated sections. The theory referred to above represents one possibility. Other models and theories meanwhile have been formulated which undoubtedly provide additional inspiration and ideas in this respect.

Are the shortcuts referred to above in our measurement of childbearing preferences and/or intentions also pitfalls ? To a certain extent they certainly are. At the same time, we find ourselves comparable to the work of most of our colleagues. Each empirical research necessarily makes concessions, as each model is necessarily based on one or more assumptions. Our concessions are mainly imposed by the vehicle carrying our research efforts: a large-scale survey involving several thousands of respondents.

Many questions remain. One of these is, how to reconcile the need for expanded data collection to suit increasingly complex models and theories, on the one hand, and on the other hand the necessity to substantially reduce the data collection costs of large-scale surveys in the domain of reproductive behaviour ?

MOTIVATION OF REPRODUCTIVE BEHAVIOUR AND THE PROFESSIONAL MOTIVATION OF WOMEN

Erika Spieß, Friedemann W. Nerdinger & Lutz von Rosenstiel
Institut für Psychologie der Universität München
Wirtschafts- und Organisationspsychologie
Leopoldstraße 13
8000 MÜNCHEN 40
Germany

6.1. Introduction

The decision by women with children to be active on the labour market is determined, to a large extent, by the preferences of the woman and her partner. This paper pays special attention to professional motivation, on the one hand, and to the desire to have children, on the other hand. Using survey data for young married women, the relation between professional activities and the desire for children is examined further and reported on in this chapter.

6.1.1. Professional motivation of women and fertility : a conflict ?

In the headlines of the West German newspapers, the employment of women has been cited as a cause of the declining birth rate. This, however, only reflects part of the problem. From the population science point of view, it has been demonstrated by Schwarz (1981) that the declining birth rate had its origin 100 years ago, whereas the employment of women has only increased since the 1960s. The participation of women in the work force requires a differentiated point of view, since it is determined by various factors. For example, the salary plays a part: if the husband has a low income, the wife will work even if they have several children, whereas wives whose husbands have a high income are employed to a lesser extent (Tegtmeyer, 1976; Von Rosenstiel et al., 1986).

Although the employment of women has become more and more self-evident, it is still burdened with several specific problems. The income of women is on average lower than that of men. Women are, to an unproportional extent, employed in jobs with little or no qualification or have part-time jobs. These positions are the ones threatened the most by unemployment. There are hardly any women in leadership and top management positions; only in the service sector does one see women in middle management (cf. Stutenbäumer-Hübner, 1985; Spieß, 1988).

There are various explanations for this, which take into account the individual motivation of women as well as the societal causes. Obsolete sex-role stereotypes and socialization effects (Lehr, 1984) are included here, as well as the societal and political causes, which cause the professional motivation of women and fertility to come into conflict. If women feel responsible for the family, the raising of children and the household, then this automatically indicates that there is less willingness and readiness for their profession (Beck-Gernsheim, 1984). In our achievement-oriented professional world, this means that women will have less advancement opportunities. The conflict for women arises from the motives to commit oneself to one's profession and the motives to have children (Scanzoni, 1978; Inglehart, 1979; Kahn-Hut *et al.*, 1982).

6.1.2. Motives for working

Organizational psychologists (Von Rosenstiel, 1987) have described several classifications of work motives. A relatively simple differentiation of the various work motives classifies them into three categories.

First, there is the "normative aspect", which means that we are expected to work. In our society there are still different expectations for men and for women. For men it is a self-evident necessity; for women the work role has also become self-evident, but not to the same degree as with men.

Second, work provides rewards (income) beyond the action itself. This means that work motivation can be extrinsic.

Third, there are also incentives within the work itself. Here the organizational psychologists speak of intrinsic motivation. The change of values which has been taking place in western industrial nations also affects the work motivation (Noelle-Neumann and Strümpel, 1984). An important result of the data analysis of Inglehart's (1977) representative survey (see also Klages and Kmieciak, 1979; Von Rosenstiel and Stengel, 1987) was that younger groups of individuals tended to have post-materialistic values. This indicates that these individuals find values such as self-actualization and environmental protection very important, while the older generation prefers materialistic values such as a high standard of living and security. Inglehart (1989) demonstrated, on the basis of cohort analysis, that the effects, for the most part, are due to differences between generations and not to ageing. However, the changing values caused by the generation change proceed very slowly. But since the post-

materialistic individuals have a better education than those who are materialistic, Inglehart supposes that these people will have a greater amount of
influence in the future. They place high expectations on their work, which fits
to this value orientation.

Due to the changing of values, women do not only want to add a financial
contribution to the family by working, they also want to fulfill and satisfy
their own needs. A survey done by Becker-Schmidt (1981), which covered the work
experiences of women in the factory and in the family, showed that the work,
even though it was experienced as being monotonous, did more than just fulfill
their extrinsic needs (financial), but also served their intrinsic needs, such
as maintaining contacts and exchanges. This displacement of motives which arose
from the changing of values gains meaning for the motivation of reproductive
behaviour.

6.1.3. Motives for having children

There have been many attempts to assess the reasons for wanting to have
children: one wants to live on through one's children, one searches for new
experiences, one likes to stabilize one's own status as an adult and one's
identity. There are, however, also *norms*, based on religion or family tradition, which influence the desire to have children (see Hoffman, 1978). In a
small pilot study in Bavaria (Büchl *et al.*, 1979), 50 women with children
were asked whether they desired a third child. Those who wanted one more child
mentioned "joy in children" as the most important reason for children, while
those who did not want anymore children said that children "belong to
marriage." One could call the "joy in children" intrinsically motivated,
whereas one could describe the attitude that children "belong to marriage" as
being steered by norms. Through the change in values, the problem for women
can only get worse, since the values for self-actualization could increase the
expectations of one's own lifestyle and decrease the desire to have a child.

The study "Changing values and reproductive behaviour", sponsored during
the years 1978-1983 by the Volkswagen Foundation, investigated the psychological causes of the declining birthrate in the Federal Republic of Germany
under the perspective of changing values. The question concerning the effect
of changing values on reproductive behaviour of women was also included.

Figure 1. A couple-interaction model of reproductive behaviour.

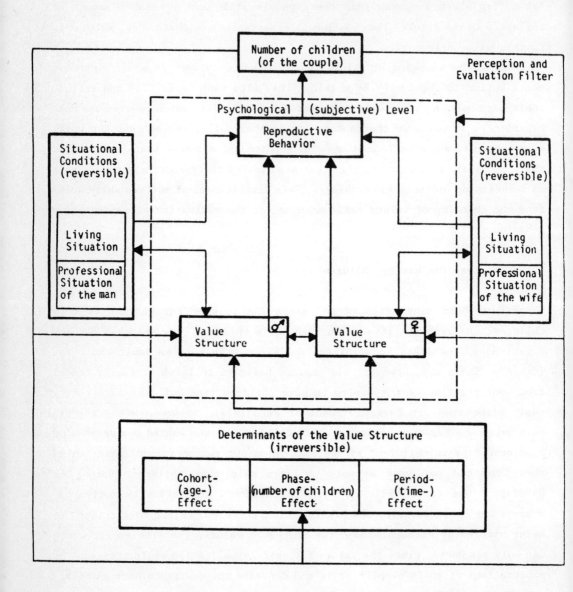

Source: Von Rosenstiel *et al.*, 1986.

6.2. The model of the study: changing values and reproductive behaviour

The goals of the study "Changing values and reproductive behaviour" were:

- the observation of the motivation for reproductive behaviour with the changing values in society as the background;
- longitudinal evaluations on a large number of married couples in Germany;
- the inclusion of men and women (husbands and wives) together in the survey.

The model of this study takes as a basis a couple model, which was developed from the study "Motivation of reproductive behaviour" (Von Rosenstiel *et al.*, 1986). Figure 1 clarifies the central themes of the study. The starting point is the individual value structure of the husband and the wife.

The "couple-interaction-model" presupposes that the values to which a person is oriented are tangible on the level of the individual and are meaningful for concrete behaviour. This means that values are transferred to an individual by the socialization process. These values serve as orientation points in different situations and determine one's behaviour and actions. Values, however, are formed and changed via a societal process. At this point the thesis of changing values in society (Inglehart, 1977; Noelle-Neumann, 1978; Klages, 1984) becomes relevant for this study.

Furthermore, the value structure includes the intrinsic values, meaning the love of children and normative aspects. This value structure is affected by irreversible determinants such as the cohort, the phase and the period effect, as well as by reversible conditions such as the living situation and the employment situation of the woman. The value structure further also affects the reversible, situational conditions and the reproductive behaviour. The irreversible conditions will now be further described.

1. *Cohort or age effect*. This means that different cohorts of couples will experience different external conditions. With these, they develop specific values and could become the age-group cohorts and central promoters of the changing of values (Ryder, 1965). For example, individuals who were born in the Federal Republic of Germany during the "building-up phase" - the period following the Second World War (1945-1955) - grew up under completely different economic and social conditions

than those who were born between 1955 and 1965, when the standard of living was higher. This affects those values that are concerned with marriage and family as well. The changing of values explained by Inglehart (1977) can be examined with the analysis of this effect.

2.   *Phase or number of children effect.* Human beings go through specific life phases from birth to death, such as starting school, entry into professional life, birth of the first child, retirement. These can be characterized by a typical role constellation. In each of these phases the life situation changes and requires a change in roles, which can also affect the values. In the longitudinal study, we are examining the birth of the first child and the birth of further children in relation to these values.

3.   *Period or time effect.* Specific occurrences affect all age groups at the same time and affect the values of all involved. For example, the hypothesis that a economic depression could change and modify values would fit into this category.

6.3. The design of the study

The study "Changing values and reproductive behaviour" was planned as a panel. The first survey took place in 1980 with 667 married couples. The sample was drawn through a multiple step random choice process of selection from the files of the justices of the peace. Subjects were selected from one large, one mid-size and one small city, as well as one rural county. The wedding date of the subjects was between 1972 and 1979. The wives were born between 1949 and 1959 and both partners were German citizens. Most families had either no child or one child at the point of questioning. A few couples had two or three children. In 1982 the second survey took place; 371 of the couples were willing to take part. Simultaneously, a control group sample of 170 couples was questioned in order to determine interview/survey effects. 539 couples participated in the third survey, including 108 couples from the first survey, 125 from the control group, the remaining 296 couples having been interviewed three times. Both partners were questioned separately at first and then together, according to the "Y-Design."

Comparisons with the official statistics indicates that the sample is representative of married couples in the Federal Republic of Germany. The only deviant factor is religion, where the Bavarian majority clearly dominated: 70% of the subjects are Catholic. This could indicate a bias in our sample. It is assumed (Fürstenberg and Mörth, 1979; Inglehart, 1989), that with the increased secularization of religion in its institutional form, it is not possible to make conclusive statements about basic religiosity. It does not seem to play a role in reproductive behaviour. (Religiosity was assessed as a value in our study. Most respondents rated it as unimportant.) Most of the individuals in the sample rent apartments, have completed secondary school and an apprentice-ship. According to the classification scheme of Kleining and Moore (1968), most of the individuals belong to the lower middle class.

6.4. Results of the study

Central to the couple-interaction-model is the individual value structure, which is determined by irreversible and reversible conditions. These will be analysed in greater detail in the following.

6.4.1. Values of reproductive behaviour

In order to assess the individual value structure, 24 value items were developed. These describe concrete life goals and are to be rated on a scale ranging from absolutely unimportant (0) to extremely important (5). Table 1 shows the important values that have been found to be the basic constructs. This value structure was replicated throughout the three periods of measure-ment, as well as with the control group.

The evaluation of the co-variation of the value orientation with the desire for children resulted (cf. Von Rosenstiel *et al.*, 1986; Spieß *et al.*, 1984; Nerdinger *et al.*, 1984) in values such as "emotional provisions for old age", "leisure" and "religion" as being important for the desire for children, rather than primarily materialistic considerations.

Table 1. The main values in the first and second enquiry.

Values	Example
Affluence	To earn a high salary
Religiosity	To live a religious life
Provisions for old age	Not to be alone in old age
Partnership	To live with one's partner in harmony
Profession	One's own professional advancement
Leisure	Frequently go to the theatre or cinema

6.4.2. Effects of age, number of children and the wish for children

The evaluation of the cohort effect indicated that young women (women who were born between 1953 and 1960) without children or with one child have a stronger wish for children than older women who were born between 1945 and 1952. The younger women also displayed a greater emotional kindness to children. This result was only partially interpreted as a confirmation of Inglehart's theory, since love for children can be interpreted as belonging to the post-materialistic values. However, the values concerning a high standard of living and leisure, which are materialistic values, seem to be important to the subjects as well.

The results of the phase-effect evaluation (defined by the number of children) resulted in a significant negative co-variation for the value area "Profession." These women in our sample clearly represented the traditional role stereotype, which states that it is inappropriate to have a profession if one has several children. Table 2 shows the wish for children of husbands and wives who have had their first child in the meantime (between 1980 and 1982), compared to those who have not had a child. The wish for children decreases in the wives and husbands who have not had a child, whereas it increases in those who have had a child in the meantime. This was evaluated as a contradiction of the so-called "Babyshock-Thesis" of Jürgens and Pohl (1975). Their study determined a decrease in the (further) wish for children in young couples after the birth of their first child.

Table 2. Desire for children 1980 and 1982 of couples childless in 1980.

child born between 1980-1982	women			men		
	1980	1982	sign.	1980	1982	sign.
no child born	1.57	1.36	*	1.53	1.42	
child born	1.89	2.22	*	1.86	2.18	*

* = p < .05 (t-test)

The evaluation of the period effect, the changes in the value structure that do not occur due to age or number of children, indicated only for women a decrease in meaning for the values "Profession" and "Leisure", that is, women found these values less important. This was interpreted as an expression of a role conflict for women who are faced with the problem of combining profession with family.

6.4.3. Job-orientation of women and the wish for children

Situation effects could affect the individual value structure (see Figure 1). However, in comparison with the irreversible determinants, the living situation and the employment of women, for example, are reversible. It is possible for women who are not satisfied with their professional situation to find a new purpose in life by fulfilling the housewife and mother role. In the same fashion, a satisfying professional life could reinforce the career preferences.

In our study the perceptions regarding the employment of women (wives) were taken into special consideration (Spieß, 1984). Table 3 displays the differences between the perceptions of the spouses regarding the reasons for the employment of women. The women were to rank these items for their professional work (the housewives their housework) on a scale ranging from 5 (applies) to 0 (does not apply). The men also were to rank the items for the work of their wives.

Table 3. Differences in the evaluation of the reasons for the housweork or the
professional work of the wife, by sex (survey 1982).

Reasons for the woman being a housewife (N = 162)	Housewife about herself	Housewife's husband about his wife	significant
The woman's wish	3.4 (1.9)	3.1 (2.1)	
The husband's wish	3.0 (2.0)	2.9 (2.1)	
A mutual decision	3.9 (1.7)	4.1 (1.6)	
It was self-evident	3.4 (1.9)	2.9 (2.1)	*
She could not find work	0.5 (1.3)	0.4 (2.1)	

Reasons for the woman being employed (N = 355)	Employed woman about herself	Employed woman's husband about his wife	significant
The woman's wish	4.4 (1.2)	4.1 (1.5)	*
The husband's wish	1.7 (1.9)	1.9 (1.8)	
A mutual decision	2.5 (2.2)	2.4 (2.1)	
It was self-evident	3.7 (1.8)	2.8 (2.1)	*
It was financially necessary	2.7 (2.0)	2.4 (1.9)	*

Standard deviation in brackets
* = $p < .05$ (t-test)

The wives rate their employment as representing the wish of the women themselves slightly higher than the men do. Second place is the item "It is self-
evident that women work", ranked much higher by wives than by husbands,
followed by the financial necessity. (The results for housewives showed that
this status is much less desired by the women.) This was interpreted to state
that the employment of women is an important value decision for the wife.

Table 4 shows the differences in the evaluation of the professional work
or housework. Housewives and employed wives differ significantly with regard
to the evaluation of their work. In all cases the employed women find their
work more interesting, more useful in maintaining contacts, more fulfilling
and more rewarding than the housewives. The sex-specific perception is interesting here: consistently the men evaluate the employed women's activity as
less interesting and fulfilling; instead, strenuousness and over-work are in
the foreground. It is possible that a tendential dissatisfaction with the

role of the woman as wife (in the eyes of the woman herself) or high demands or expectations that the husband has of the wife could explain this.

Furthermore, it was possible to determine differences in the value struc-ture of the housewives and the employed wives. The housewives had a stronger religious orientation, while the employed women placed more importance

Table 4. Differences in the evaluation of the professional work or of the housework of wife, by sex (survey 1982).

Evaluation of housework (N = 162)	Housewife about herself	Housewife's husband about his wife	significant
She has interesting work	2.5 (1.6)	2.6 (1.5)	
She has a large amount of contact with people	2.6 (1.6)	2.6 (1.5)	
She is bound to set working hours	1.1 (1.5)	1.4 (1.6)	
She feels overworked	1.2 (1.4)	1.7 (1.5)	*
Her work is strenuous	2.0 (1.6)	3.4 (1.4)	*
During work she can speak to her family	4.2 (1.2)	4.0 (1.2)	
Her work fulfills her	3.1 (1.6)	3.1 (1.6)	
Her work is recognized	3.6 (1.4)	4.0 (1.1)	*
Evaluation of professional work (N = 355)	Employed woman about herself	Employed woman's husband about his wife	significant
She has interesting work	3.9 (1.3)	3.7 (1.3)	*
She has a large amount of contact with people	4.1 (1.3)	4.0 (1.4)	
She is bound to set working hours	3.3 (2.1)	3.4 (1.9)	
She feels overworked	1.4 (1.4)	1.7 (1.5)	*
Her work is strenuous	2.9 (1.6)	3.3 (1.3)	*
During work she can speak to her family	2.6 (1.9)	2.6 (1.8)	
Her work fulfills her	3.7 (1.3)	3.5 (1.3)	*
Her work is recognized	4.1 (1.1)	4.1 (1.1)	

Standard deviation in brackets
* = p < .05 (t-test)

on the "Profession" and "Leisure" values. The following question arises: are the value orientations the result of the decision to work solely in the household or to be employed ? Are the values adapted to the actual situation or do they determine the decisions ?

In order to investigate this issue, new groups were formed: housewives who retained this status in 1982 were compared with housewives who became employed by 1982, as well as employed women in 1980 who then became housewives by 1982 with employed women who retained this status in 1982 (Table 5).

The results indicate that housewives who remained true to their status, as well as employed wives who became housewives, tended to have more conservative values than wives who remained employed or became employed (again). A discriminant analytic examination of the data was able to confirm the importance of the values for the occupational status of the woman: in 70% of the cases it was possible to correctly predict the woman's occupational status according to the value orientation in 1980. If women tended to have more

Table 5. Values according to professional status, 1982.

Value 1980	Employed who remained employed	Employed who became housewives	significant
Affluence	2.9 (0.9)	3.3 (0.9)	*
Religiosity	1.4 (1.5)	1.9 (1.3)	*
Provisions for old age	4.0 (1.0)	4.3 (1.0)	
Partnership	4.7 (0.4)	4.9 (0.2)	*
Profession	3.8 (0.9)	3.4 (1.1)	*
Leisure	2.6 (1.0)	2.4 (0.9)	
Value 1980	Housewives who remained housewives	housewives who became employed	significant
Affluence	2.9 (0.9)	2.6 (1.1)	
Religiosity	1.9 (1.3)	1.7 (1.5)	
Provisions for old age	4.2 (0.8)	4.3 (0.9)	
Partnership	4.8 (0.4)	4.8 (0.5)	
Profession	2.9 (0.9)	3.4 (1.0)	*
Leisure	2.1 (1.0)	2.5 (1.1)	

Standard deviation in brackets
* = p < .05 (t-test)

religious and emotional values, they were more likely to give up their profession. This group also had significantly more children in 1982.

A path analytic examination of the relationship between professional orientation and the desire to have children (Figure 2) showed that the desire to have children influences the woman's professional orientation: the greater the desire to have children at the first point of questioning, the lower the professional orientation at the second point of questioning (Nerdinger, 1984). The fact that the professional orientation of women is influenced by the desire to have children leads us to consider the specific socialization conditions of women, as well as the restrictive conditions and opportunities of society regarding reproductive behaviour. However, whether a couple decides to have children or not is also a question of their personal lifestyle and their entire value structure. This value structure also includes the concept of female employment.

Figure 2. Causal dependence between profession and total desire for children (TDC)

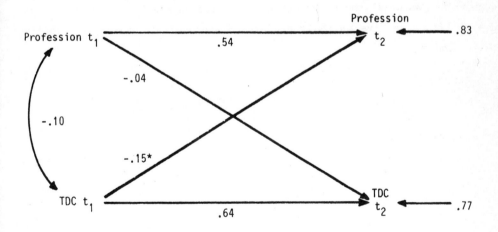

6.5. Conclusion

The professional life of women and the wish to have children presents a conflict between two motives: the motive to be professionally active and the motive to have children. This conflict has become more extreme under the influence of a societal changing of values: young women, in particular, place higher demands on their lifestyle. However, their expectations of professional life have also increased: women do not only want to earn a little bit extra for the family, but also want to become fulfilled by their work.

The study "Changing values and reproductive behaviour" demonstrates, using a sample of young married women, that values are of great importance for reproductive behaviour. The wish for children is determined by values such as "leisure" and "emotional provisions for old age care", whereas the value "profession" correlates negatively with the number of children. If one interprets the results using the "preferences-restrictions-behaviour scheme", the value "profession" is an obstacle for women who have a high wish for children. The other way round, children hinder a pronounced professional motivation. If women are driven by the preference "profession" or "professional career", then they will most likely decide against having children. Preferences are expressed through values as well: those who place high value on emotional and religious values will tend to give up their profession and dedicate themselves wholly to their family.

A PURPOSEFUL BEHAVIOUR THEORY OF WORK AND FAMILY SIZE DECISIONS

Richard P. Bagozzi
Graduate School of Business Administration
University of Michigan
ANN ARBOR, Michigan 48109-1234
U.S.A.

M. Frances Van Loo
School of Business Administration
University of California at Berkeley
BERKELEY, California 94720
U.S.A.

7.1. Introduction

Our goal in this chapter will be to develop a theory of work and family size decisions at the level of the social psychology of a man and woman in an intimate relationship. Four assumptions shape the form and substance of our theory. Firstly, we assume that work and family size considerations must be integrated in any valid theory and that these considerations function as either simultaneous or sequential criteria (Bagozzi and Van Loo, 1988; Van Loo and Bagozzi, 1984). By simultaneous criteria we mean that work and family size decisions are decided upon contemporaneously in either explicit or implicit choice processes. This might occur at one point in time such as at the outset of marriage but more likely than not happens intermittently throughout the course of the relationship. By sequential criteria we mean that one or the other are decided upon with the alternative functioning as either a pre-existing or anticipated constraint.

A second assumption we make is that work and family size decisions are both motivated and reasoned (Bagozzi and Van Loo, 1990). By motivated we mean that the decisions are goal-directed and that emotional factors play a role. By reasoned we mean that judgments are made of the likelihood and evaluation of the consequences of action or inaction and that choices are made both among alternative goals and among means to achieve the goals.

Thirdly, we presume that work and family size decisions are made at least partly in response to the social environment in which they are embedded (Bagozzi and Van Loo, 1980; 1987, pp. 198-199). This manifests itself in two ways: as normative pressure from society at large and as interpersonal give and take among family members and between the partners in a relationship and significant others outside the family.

Finally, our theory is based on the premise that the fullest explanations of work and family size decisions rest on specification of the elementary psychological processes going on within the bodies and minds of men and women and the social psychological processes transpiring between them as they socially construct their life experiences. Many theories in the social sciences have ignored these processes by focussing only upon the associations between inputs (e.g. income, education) and outputs (e.g. employment, family size). Our aim is the develop a theory specifying the intervening mechanisms.

To do this, we draw heavily upon basic research in the psychology and social psychology literatures. Because these literatures have evolved in rather piecemeal ways and have only addressed portions of the underlying processes in work and family size decisions, we have had to revise and integrate a number of leading contemporary theories into our framework. In the process, we have discovered a number of omissions in the literature which necessitated the formulation of new thinking that better reflects the idiosyncrasies in work and family size decisions. Thus our theory is in part a synthesis and extension of other theories and in part a development of new ideas.

7.2. Overview of theory

Figure 1 presents an outline of our theory. The focal point is the goal(s) one has or the outcome(s) one experiences. A goal is a desired end state or action, while an outcome is something that happens or accrues to oneself, either desired or not. For example, having a child is a goal if it is planned, an outcome if not. Planning for an early retirement is a goal, while an unexpected discharge from work is an outcome.

With respect to end states, one may either experience or anticipate an outcome, choose a goal from among a set of goals, or simply "have" a goal. These are shown in figure 1 as paths a, b, and c, respectively. The experience or anticipation of an outcome leads to subjective expected utility reactions toward the consequences of the outcome (path a). In contrast, assuming that one has weighed the subjective expected utilities of the implications of achieving multiple goals (path b), one or more goals may be chosen for actual pursuit and the means for goal achievement considered (path d). Finally, rather than choosing a goal from among others, per se, one might on occassion seek a single goal uncritically. This occurs, for example, when one spontaneously feels the need to have a child (as a function of biological and/or emotional forces, say) and accepts this, temporarily at least, as his or her goal. It also occurs when social forces, felt moral duty, habit, or impulse impose themselves on one's will in a singular fashion. Thus path c in figure 1 reflects the impact of a singular goal on one's subjective expected utility reactions toward the consequences of goal achievement or failure to achieve the goal. Note that, although the acceptance of a singular goal can be more or less automatic, the way it is manifested and elaborated upon is very much a reasoned process.

The remaining paths in figure 1 and their accompanying components address the social psychological reactions toward or in relation to singular goals. We can think of each goal in a set of possible goals as eliciting its own set of components parallel to those shown in figure 1. The choice among goals, if indeed a choice is to be made, involves comparisons of the consequences of each goal and selection of one or more goals according to some decision rule. We will return to the problem of goal choice later in the chapter. For now, we wish to consider the remainder of the processes outlined in figure 1 which refer to the psychological meaning of and motives for goal pursuit and the decision processes leading to the choice of means.

The implications of goal achievement or failure to achieve a goal are particularistic and rather concrete. Having a child leads to feelings of joy, amusing experiences, companionship, lost sleep, financial costs, and family stress. Working leads to economic resources, professional fulfillment, friendships, anxiety, loss of free time, and job stress. The subjective expected utilities of these specific consequences achieve meaning in a phenomenological sense when they become transformed into more global psychological responses (path e in figure 1). Affective reactions toward successfully achieving a goal or failing to do so constitute one type of higher order psychological response in this sense. That is, expectations and evaluations of individual consequences of goal/outcome attainment become integrated and produce multiple emotional responses toward success and toward failure. Similarly, overall affective responses toward the process of trying to achieve a goal (as opposed to the consequences of success or failure) are another type of higher order emotional reaction. For instance, trying to have a child might involve considerable planning and effort with respect to the monitoring of ovulation, the timing of intercourse, trips to the doctor, and so on. In addition to affective responses, higher order psychological reactions arise in the form of global cognitive representations. Particularly meaningful here are judgments about the likelihood that one's goal directed behaviours will succeed or fail (i.e., one's self-efficacy).

Social processes are represented in the theory through felt normative pressure (path g). The perceived expectations of significant others and one's motivation to comply with these expectations comprise the primary variables representing the effects of social processes (cf. Van Loo and Bagozzi, 1984).

Affective, self-efficacy, and normative processes are the direct impetuses for decisions concerning how to pursue a goal (paths f and g in figure 1). Recall also that a choice process among means can be activated after a choice of a goal has been made from among alternatives (path d). The volitional part of decision making with respect to means involves assessments of the specific self-efficacies for individual instrumental actions, the likelihood that these actions would lead to goal achievement, one's liking/disliking of the actions, and the psychological commitment and amount of effort one is willing to put forth in the initiation of one or more of the actions. The choice part of decision making entails a comparison of alternative instrumental actions and selection of one or more according to a rule. One's choice is then expressed as an intention to act (e.g. a goal to have a child might stimulate intentions to take fertility drugs and increase the frequency of intercourse; a goal to pursue a career might lead to intentions to visit an employment agency, take a public speaking course, and prepare a new resume).

Intentions, in turn, are directed toward actual initiation of one or more instrumental acts (path h in figure 1) which then leads to goal achievement (path i), assuming that conditions are favourable. The ability of an instrumental act to produce its effects is conditioned on facilitating or inhibiting forces in the situation. These forces might be physical, biological, economic, temporal, or social in nature. Some forces interact with instrumental acts to influence goal/outcome attainment (path j), others directly influence goal/-outcome attainment (path k). An example of an interaction effect would be the conjunction of emotional stress inhibiting conception with a couple's planned efforts to have a child. An example of a direct facilitating effect would be a windfall promotion on the job which produces an increment in one's work aspirations.

Figure 1. Outline of purposeful behaviour theory of work and family size decisions.

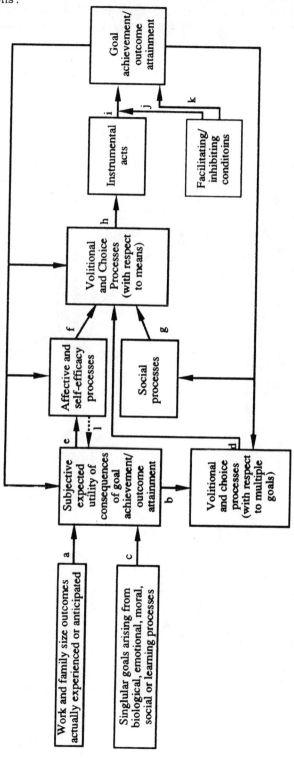

Figure 2. Illustration of a multidimensional expectancy-value model toward
          "having children".
          (Boxes encompass concrete expectancy-value responses, circles and
          ellipses represent higher order psychological abstractions).

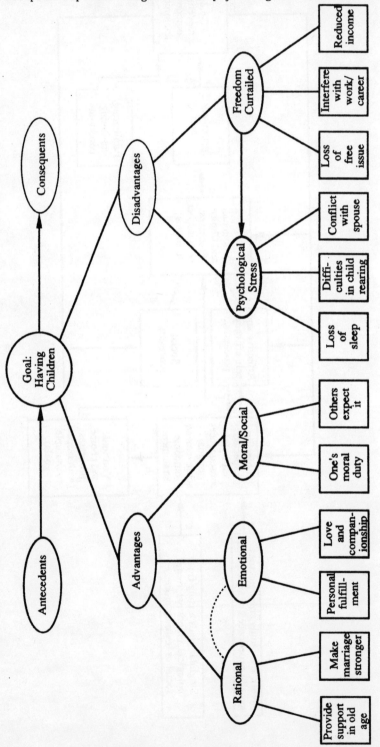

Once one achieves a goal or experiences an outcome, feedback occurs upon each of the social psychological processes shown in figure 1. We turn now to a more detailed specification of the components and subprocesses comprising the theory.

7.3. The consequences of goal achievement/outcome attainment

People anticipate or experience the consequences of achieving a goal or failing to do so as beliefs (b_i) about the likelihood of occurrence of the consequences, and evaluations (e_i) of the desirability or noxiousness of these consequences. Example b_i's for work include the perceived likelihood that work will lead to financial security, feeling fulfilled, and less time for family (e.g. Sperber *et al.* 1980, p. 125). Example b_i's for family size decisions are the perceived likelihood that having children would result in a lowered standard of living, enhanced feelings of being loved and needed, and less personal time (e.g. Vinokur-Kaplan, 1977). The b_i's are measured on bipolar likely/unlikely scales or on subjective probability indices. The e_i's are generally measured on bipolar semantic differential scales (e.g. good/bad indices). The integration of these reactions are typically expressed as the $\Sigma b_i e_i$ and have been termed subjective expected utility (e.g. Edwards, 1961) or expectancy-value attitudes (e.g. Ajzen and Fishbein, 1980; Fishbein and Ajzen, 1975) in the literature. Because a large body of research can be found applying the approach to both fertility (e.g. Davidson and Jaccard, 1975; Vinokur-Kaplan, 1978) and work (e.g. Sperber *et al.*, 1980) settings, we will limit discussion here to shortcomings and extensions of expectancy-value theory.

7.3.1. The functional form of expectancy-value reactions

The form of the $\Sigma b_i e_i$, while intuitive, is rather simplistic. Some work has been done specifying alternative functional forms including cases where beliefs and evaluations combine in linear and nonlinear ways, beliefs and evaluations serve as indicators of latent psychological reactions, beliefs and evaluations function as complex determinants of psychological constructs, and other variations (e.g. Bagozzi, 1985). To date, none of these developments has been applied in fertility or work contexts, but they offer opportunities for better modelling how beliefs and evaluations a) are organized in human memory,

b) change in response to new information and persuasive communications, and
c) influence preferences and choice.

7.3.2. Multidimensional expectancy-value reactions

Related to the functional form of expectancy-value reactions is the issue of
dimensionality. The traditional model assumes an unidimensional response
(i.e., a singular summary of one's beliefs and evaluations organized as the
sum of corresponding products). A multidimensional alternative has been
suggested in the psychology literature consisting of separate expectancy-value
reactions represented through a pattern or hierarchy of interconnected belief
times evaluation terms (e.g. Bagozzi, 1981a, 1981b, 1990a).

Figure 2 presents a hypothetical example of an expectancy-value structural
hierarchy applied to the goal of "having children." At the top is the most
general or abstract representation(s), in this case the notion of having
children as a global idea in memory. At the bottom are the more concrete
responses which consist of the products of individual beliefs times evaluations
(e.g. the perceived likelihood that having children will lead to a stronger
marriage multiplied by one's felt importance or need for a stronger marriage).
The concrete responses shown in the boxes are actual measurements of people's
cognitions and evaluations and may be obtained as self-reports on a questionnaire, psychophysiological reactions (e.g. electromyogram readings of facial
muscles; electroencephalogram monitoring of cortical brain activity), or
behavioural observations by a trained observer.

In the middle of figure 2 are displayed psychological constructs at
intermediate levels of abstraction. For the particular example shown, two
higher level abstractions are represented - advantages and disadvantages -
which represent aggregations or summary abstractions of more specific
expectancy-value responses. Below the higher level abstractions can be found
five lower level abstractions which are nonoverlapping special cases (e.g.
emotional advantages, psychological stress). Thus a total of four levels exist
for this particular example, each linked hierarchically and organized from the
most abstract at the top to the most concrete at the bottom. Straight line
segments are used to express hierarchical linkages. These linkages constitute
logical or categorical relations among higher levels, and correspondence rules
between the lowest level and adjacent higher level variables. The number,
nature, and organization of abstract categories depend on basic storage

processes in human memory. Note further that relations among concepts within a particular level of the hierarchy may be correlative or causal. For instance, rational and emotional advantages might be positively associated in a decision maker's mind (see dashed arc in figure 2). Similarly, the curtailment of one's freedom might lead to psychological stress (see arrow in figure 2). The latter could be a perceived causal connection or an inference process within the mind of a decision maker.

Structures such as that shown in figure 2 can be used to represent expectancy-value reactions as they are actually stored in memory and obviously contain more information than the oversimplified $\Sigma b_i e_i$. Theory development can be more precise as well, in that hypotheses are represented as linkages among abstract variables and these are tied, in turn, to less abstract variables and ultimately to concrete observations in one integrated system. Such a framework has received considerable attention in the social sciences of late, and attempts have been made to ground the approach in philosophy of science criteria (e.g. Bagozzi, 1984a). Structural equation models with latent variables can be used to formally implement such theoretical frameworks.

A number of benefits of the multidimensional expectancy-value conceptual-izaton should be pointed out. The $\Sigma b_i e_i$ is a rather course-grained representation of human judgment processes and indeed emphasizes prediction more than it does explanation. When we relate expectancy-value reactions to their antecedents and consequents within the body of a larger theory, the use of a multidimensional representation permits one to model the differential dependencies, and implications, of distinct expectancy-value components. For example, it might be the case that child preferences for some couples are driven primarily by rational considerations whereas for other couples by emotional and moral factors. The $\Sigma b_i e_i$ captures the total effects of separate expectancy-value responses but does not provide for the identification of the particular sources of these effects. The multidimensional representation provides a decomposition of individual expectancy-value responses and can, within the context of structural equation models with latent variables (e.g. Bagozzi, 1981a, 1990a), yield fine-grained explanations contingent on distinct expectancy-value functions.

In addition to its explanatory role in theory development and testing, multidimensional expectancy-value representations provide pragmatic and policy benefits. From a diagnostic point of view, multidimensional representations can be used in exploratory or descriptive senses to aid in pretesting, questionnaire design, and reliability and validity assessment (e.g. Bagozzi, 1981b). From a normative perspective, multidimensional expectancy-value models can suggest which beliefs and/or evaluations are more susceptible to change (and thus point to fruitful targets in education campaigns) and which beliefs and evaluations are predictive of or influential in attitude and behaviour change, thereby informing forecasts and providing strategic information to change agents.

7.3.3. Measurement issues

The scales of measurement of beliefs and evaluations pose special problems in empirical research but have often been ignored by social scientists who use expectancy-value models in their studies (e.g. Bagozzi, 1984b). The primary problem is that, when either beliefs or evaluations are at best measured on interval scales, an indeterminacy exists in the estimation of the effects of expectancy-value product terms. This is especially an issue in across-subjects designs and when questionnaire data are employed, which typically rest on ordinal or interval variables.

Three methodological solutions exist. Hierarchical regression overcomes the problem of scale indeterminacy but does not correct for measurement error in beliefs and evaluations (e.g. Bagozzi, 1984b). Structural equation models with latent variables and use of full information estimation procedures solve both the indeterminacy and measurement error problems but rely on assumptions of multivariate normality and large samples (e.g. Kenny and Judd, 1984). Partial least squares procedures surmount the indeterminacy and measurement error issues and at the same time are suitable for small samples and make no assumptions on the distribution of variates or scales of measurement (e.g. Bagozzi, 1990a).

Another problem peculiar to the incorporation of multidimensional expectancy-value reactions in empirical research is multicollinearity. The regression of attitudes, for example, on multiple expectancy-value reactions often results in imprecise parameter estimates and obscures the discovery of valid effects. One remedy is to use structural equation models with latent variables and regress attitudes directly on a higher order expectancy-value factor (e.g. Bagozzi, 1981a, 1981b, 1985). Because attitudes would thus be a function of a higher-order factor and the concrete measures are functions of the factor, the source of multicollinearity is eliminated.

7.3.4. A purposeful behaviour alternative

Traditionally, the motivational component of the expectancy-value model (i.e., "evaluations") has been conceived of as either an evaluative judgment or an affective reaction (e.g. Ajzen and Fishbein, 1980). To measure the component, researchers have most frequently used the good/bad bipolar semantic differential item. This practice may be satisfactory when affect and moral impetuses are congruent. But when they constitute distinct psychological responses, as happens in most work and family size decisions, it is unclear what the good/bad item is measuring.

Bagozzi (1986) recently showed that the motivational component of expectancy-value reactions is neither an affective nor moral one. Rather, affective and moral impulses are in fact antecedents to approach-avoidance tendencies which, in turn, serve as operationalizations of the motivational component. Specifically, an approach-avoidance tendency can be measured as the subjective conditional probability that one would act, given the occurrence of a particular consequence (b_i). Further, affective and moral pressure can be seen to act additively or multiplicatively to influence approach-avoidance responses, depending on the degree of involvement and the attractiveness and likelihood of anticipated consequences (Bagozzi, 1989). To date, the theory has only been applied to the decision whether to give blood or not, where it was shown to be superior in explanatory and predictive power to the traditional expectancy-value model.

7.4. Affective and self-efficacy processes

7.4.1. Affect

Expectancy-value reactions become transformed and integrated through attitude formation processes. In particular, individual expectancy-value reactions combine to produce higher order affective states in an individual. These higher order states are manifest as emergent attitudes. As an aside, we should acknowledge that attitudes sometimes feedback, or emerge first before reasoned responses, to influence subsequent expectancy-value reactions (see dashed path 1 in figure 1). This is known as the halo effect but will not be discussed further in this paper (e.g. Bagozzi, 1990b). The halo effect occurs, for instance, when one develops an attitude toward work based on classical or operant conditioning and this, in turn, colours one's beliefs and evaluations of anticipated consequences of employment.

We propose that three attitudes function in goal-directed work and family size settings. These represent one's global affective reactions toward the perceived consequences of a) trying to achieve a goal and succeeding, b) trying to achieve a goal and failing, and c) experiencing pleasant and unpleasant outcomes while engaged in the *process* of goal pursuit. For purposes of discussion, these are termed: attitudes toward success (A_s), attitudes toward failure (A_f), and attitudes toward the process of pursuing a goal (A_p). In a conceptual paper, Warshaw *et al.* (forthcoming) were the first to consider these as separate dimensions of attitudes (see also Ajzen, 1985). Bagozzi and Warshaw (1990a, 1990b) developed the theory further and provided the first empirical test of the attitudinal components which received support in both construct validity and predictive senses.

We hypothesize that men and women develop separate A_s, A_f, and A_p psychological reactions toward the concepts of trying to achieve work and family size related goals. A goal to avoid having children, for example, results in global feelings of trying to avoid pregnancy and succeeding, trying to avoid pregnancy and failing, and trying, per se, as disclosed through the process of attempting to prevent a pregnancy (e.g. attitudes toward using rhythm, birth control pills, or contraceptives). A goal to pursue a career engenders global feelings toward trying and succeeding, trying and failing, and the process required to pursue a career.

7.4.2. Self-efficacy

Before we show how A_s, A_f, and A_p function to influence decisions, it is necessary to consider the role of global cognitive responses. Self-efficacy refers to a person's assessment of whether he or she can or cannot perform a particular behaviour or achieve a specific goal. In an impressive set of studies, Bandura (1977, 1982) has shown that self-efficacy judgments mediate the effects of nearly every mode of psychological change and decision making on the initiation of action and/or goal achievement. Building on this research, it is hypothesized herein that self-efficacy judgments in fact function in separate success and failure formats. In particular, it is proposed that the impact of A_s and A_f on decisions depend, respectively, on the decision maker's expectations of success (E_s) and expectations of failure (E_f). That is, neither the desire to succeed nor the absence of a fear of failure are regarded as sufficient predictors of favourable decisions. Rather, both must be accompanied by promising anticipations of success and unlikely forecasts of failure, respectively, for these attitudes to produce their predicted effects. Note that, although the probability of success and failure logically sum to 1.00, one's E_s and E_f need not, and phenomenologically often do not, sum to 1.00 in that people frequently form distinct and only loosely connected judgments with respect to success and failure. Finally, it is important to point out that E_s and E_f are different from the b_i. Thus, E_s and E_f are, respectively, the perceived likelihood that success or failure will occur (e.g. the perceived likelihood that one will have a child or career if he or she tries), whereas the b_i refer to the perceived likelihood that specified *consequences* will result from success, failure, or trying (e.g. the perceived likelihood that if one has a child, he or she will incur considerable financial costs, or if one pursues a career, he or she will experience new stresses).

7.4.3. Integration of affect and self-efficacy

With this as a backdrop, four functional forms are hypothesized for the effects of attitudes on decisions (e.g. on intentions to try to achieve a goal, I_t). These forms result when the three attitudinal components either have additive or interactive effects and either operate as direct determinants or alternatively become transformed into an even more global, higher-order attitude toward trying to achieve a goal (A_t). The four forms can be written as (expressed in regression equations for ease of presentation):

1. Additive-decomposed attitude:

   $I_t = \alpha_1 + \beta_1 A_s E_s + \beta_2 A_f E_f + \beta_3 A_p + \epsilon_1$

2. Multiplicative-decomposed attitude:

   $I_t = \alpha_2 + \beta_1 A_s E_s A_f E_f A_p + \epsilon_2$

3. Additive-higher-order attitude:

   $A_t = \alpha_3 + \beta_1 A_s E_s + \beta_2 A_f E_f + \beta_3 A_p + \epsilon_3$

   $I_t = \alpha_4 + \beta A_t + \epsilon_4$

4. Multiplicative-higher-order attitude:

   $A_t = \alpha_5 + \beta_1 A_s E_s A_f E_f A_p + \epsilon_5$

   $I_t = \alpha_6 + \beta A_t + \epsilon_6$

where α_i and β_j are parameters to be estimated, ϵ_i are error terms, and the remaining symbols are as defined heretofore.

Forms 1 and 3 apply when success, failure, and process considerations have independent, compensatory effects on decisions. That is, only one of the attitudinal components need be high for a favourable decision to result or low for an unfavourable decision to be made. For example, one's attitude toward a career might be so positive and one's confidence in his or her abilities so high that a decision to pursue a career is made irrespective of the consequences of failure and the obstacles perceived in the way. Another individual might value work highly and not be concerned by thoughts of possible failure on the job, yet decide not to try to get a job because of the time and impediments perceived to be in the way. Forms 2 and 4, in contrast, suggest that decisions are a function of the interactions among attitudinal components. A favourable decision requires high scores on each of A_sE_s, A_fE_f, and A_p. Thus, for instance, a couple might decide to try to have children only if they value children highly, anticipate that they have a reasonable probability of achieving conception, do not feel that failure to conceive will be emotionally devastating, and find the positive aspects of the process exciting, the negative not too onerous.

The need for A_t arises when a differentiated attitude becomes unitized. This may happen when the stimulus changes from a complex to a simple entity in the mind of the decision maker (as a consequence of past or vicarious experiences, for example), when attitude becomes stored in memory as a hierarchical representation, or when cognitive consistency or other psychological mechanisms operate to push for a convergence in mental representations. Empirical work is needed into the conditions under which each of the four forms function. To date, forms 2 and 4 have not been tested. Form 1 and 3 have been tested and found to explain intentions in the context of the weight loss decision (e.g. Bagozzi and Warshaw, 1990a).

Affective and self-efficacy processes serve an intermediary role in the social psychology of decision making by functioning as moderators between subjective expected utility reactions toward specific consequences of goal achievement/outcome attainment, on the one hand, and volitional and choice processes with respect to the means for implementing goal pursuit, on the other hand (see figure 1). The linkage between subjective expected utility reactions and affective processes (path e in figure 1) occurs through the specification of functional relations between the b_ie_i and attitudes. Taking the simple sum of products as an illustration, we have the following equations: $A_s = f(\Sigma b_i e_i)$, $A_f = f(\Sigma b_j e_j)$, and $A_p = f(\Sigma b_k e_k)$ where separate beliefs and evaluations exist for each attitudinal component reflecting the unique consequences associated with success, failure, and the process of goal pursuit, respectively. When the $b_i e_i$ are organized in multidimensional structures, the functional relationships to attitudes are of course more complex. These can be expressed through systems of simultaneous equations linking latent variables and measurements but will not be discussed herein for the sake of brevity (e.g. Bagozzi, 1981a, 1981b, 1985, 1990a).

The connections between affective and self-efficacy processes on the one hand and volitional and choice processes on the other (path f in figure 1) can be specified along the lines presented heretofore for forms 1-4. However, we should stress that the intention to try to achieve a goal (I_t) is only one component of volitional and choice processes, and the linkages will frequently be more complex (cf. Bagozzi, 1990d). We will return to volitional and choice processes shortly.

A final issue we wish to raise with respect to higher order affective responses is that these need not be unidimensional emotional reactions. Attitudes toward success, failure, and the process of goal pursuit can each exist as multidimensional structures under certain conditions. This parallels research into human emotion which typically finds two-dimensional structures such as positive/negative affect (e.g. Watson and Tellegen, 1985) and pleasantness/unpleasantness arousal (e.g. Russell, 1979). Others have found different and/or more complex patterns (e.g. Boyle, 1986). For example, Bagozzi (1990c) found that attitudes toward giving blood formed as separate, yet intercorrelated, affective and instrumental responses. Similar results have been found for attitudes toward being religious (Bagozzi and Burnkrant, 1979) and attitudes toward brands of products (Batra and Ahtola, 1987). The organization of multidimensional global attitudes in memory depends on the emotional state of the person when attitudes are learned or when an existing attitude is retrieved from memory, among other factors. Bagozzi (1990c) hypothesized that emotional arousal can affect the representation of attitudes. He predicted that the association between affective and utilitarian components could be intensified through stimulation of heightened arousal. A spreading activation theory of memory was used to explain these effects (e.g. Bower, 1981). That is, the induction of arousal energizes the most affectively charged nodes in memory and then migrates to less affectively charged nodes which are interconnected semantically in the mind. In a controlled laboratory experiment, this indeed resulted where the intercorrelation between two dimensions of attitudes increased from r = .69 in a control group to near perfect association in an experimental group (p < .01). Arousal is also likely to play a role in family size and work decisions.

A limited notion of multidimensional attitudes has been investigated in the work and family size decision contexts by a number of researchers. Bagozzi and Van Loo (1987), Beckman *et al.* (1983), and Thomson (1983) considered multidimensional attitudes toward the value of children. Bagozzi and Van Loo (1988) and Van Loo and Bagozzi (1984) addressed multidimensional sex role norms and their impact on female labour force participation and family size. However, the roles of A_s, A_f, and A_p - unidimensional or otherwise - have not yet been studied empirically in the work and family size settings.

7.4.4. Social Processes

A long tradition exists in sociology treating the effects of society on work and family size decisions as normative effects (e.g. Scanzoni, 1975; Smith-Lovin and Tickamyer, 1978; Waite and Stolzenberg, 1975). However, these approaches generally consider only the cause and effect relations between the presence of norms and their presumed outcomes and do not attempt to model the mechanisms whereby norms affect decisions and choices and lead to specific actions.

In our theory, we represent social processes through their impact on felt normative pressure. We begin with Fishbein and Ajzen's (1975; Ajzen and Fishbein, 1980) concept of social norms (SN), but unlike these authors who define SN as the person's perception that most people who are important to oneself believe he or she should or should not perform a particular behaviour, we focus on SN_t, the subjective norm toward trying to achieve a goal. Note that SN incorporates felt pressure from others contingent on success or failure (e.g. "other people expect me to perform behaviour x"), whereas SN_t focusses only on felt pressure from others to get one to attempt to pursue a goal (e.g. "other people expect me to try to get a job"). The relation of social processes to volitional and choice processes (path g in figure 1) can be expressed in equation form as follows (taking only the decision to try, I_t, as a criterion, for simplicity):

$$I_t = \alpha + b_1(A_sE_s) + b_2(A_fE_f) + b_3A_p + b_4SN_t + \epsilon.$$

The felt social norm to try to pursue a goal, in turn, is hypothesized to be a function of a) the normative beliefs that particular significant others think that one should or should not try to pursue a goal (NB_i) and b) one's motivation to comply with the expectations of those significant others (MC_i). One's normative beliefs are typically measured as follows: "My [referent - e.g. parents] think that I should have another child," and are indicated on a 7-point likely/unlikely index. Similarly, one's motivation to comply is often measured as follows: "Generally speaking, I want to do what my [referent] thinks I should do", and is recorded also on a 7-point likely/unlikely index. With respect to the form of these reactions, the most common practice is to multiply the NB_i and MC_i together in order to reflect the presumed interaction between the two in influencing SN_t (i.e., NB_i and MC_i must both be high before one will feel social pressure to achieve a goal). The products so formed are then summed across a set of salient referents to yield an aggregate representation: $SN_t = f(\Sigma(NB_i)(MC_i))$. Of course, in a manner parallel to that described earlier for the expectancy-value model, the individual products of the NB_i and MC_i could be organized complexly in memory as hierarchical structures, but we will not explore this possibility here for the sake of brevity. In terms of referents, Vinokur-Kaplan (1978), for example, scrutinized six in her study of family size decisions: spouse, parents, siblings and other close family members, close friends, in-laws, and people who held the same religious or moral beliefs. In their investigation of women's occupational orientations, Sperber *et al.* (1980) considered nine referents: mother, father, close friends, boyfriend, pastor, school counselor, teachers, career women, and housewives.

In sum, we have represented social processes through their internalization by the person undergoing decision making activities. This is primarily a psychological point of view. It should be acknowledged that social processes can also be represented as interpersonal activities, but these have not as yet been incorporated into our theory (cf. Bagozzi and Van Loo, 1980, 1987; Beckman, 1979).

7.5. Volitional processes

Affective, self-efficacy, and social processes are the direct impetuses for
making choices among means to pursue a goal and for making commitments and
forming specific intentions to implement instrumental actions directed toward
goal achievement. Figure 3 outlines the major volitional and choice processes
occurring before the actual initiation of instrumental acts. The process begins
with a consideration of alternative means for goal pursuit. This might involve
retrieval from memory of a set of means previously used or the generation of
a new set. The process might be spontaneous and unplanned or it might be
purposefully driven. Normative guidelines exist, too, such as found in
Etzioni's (1967, p. 286) mixed-scanning strategy and Janis and Mann's (1977)
model of decision making. For example, a person with a goal to pursue a career
might consider such means as the practising of job interviews, preparation of
a new resume, researching firms, and working through an employment agency.

Given a set of alternative means, three assessment processes are proposed
for appraising the means preliminary to making a choice among them. One of
these is termed specific self-efficacies of means. For each alternative, a
decision maker is hypothesized to make a subjective judgment of his or her
ability to implement the act. For example, a person deciding to pursue a
career might assess, implicitly or explicitly, his or her confidence that one
can successfully perform each of the actions thought necessary.

A second assessment process concerns the judgement that a given action
will lead to goal attainment. We have labelled these instrumentalities in
figure 3. Bandura (1977) terms these outcome expectancies. Thus, to take again
the example of pursuit of a career as a goal, it is hypothesized that decision
makers perform subjective judgments of the likelihood that each of a set of
means will lead to achievement of a specific career (e.g. the perceived
probability that making personal contacts will contribute to finding a job).

The final assessment process captures one's emotional reactions to the
means. Each alternative path toward a goal will engender different levels of
liking/disliking, pleasantness/unpleasantness, or attraction/repulsion. We
propose that a decision maker has a separate affective response to each of a
set of alternative means for goal pursuit. These might be strictly emotional
such as found in a "gut reaction" or spontaneous expression of joy or disgust
or they might be a mixture of affect and thought such as reflected in reasoned
evaluations of a favourable/unfavourable or pro/con type.

Figure 3. Outline of major decision making components and processes related to choices among means and the initiation of instrumental acts.

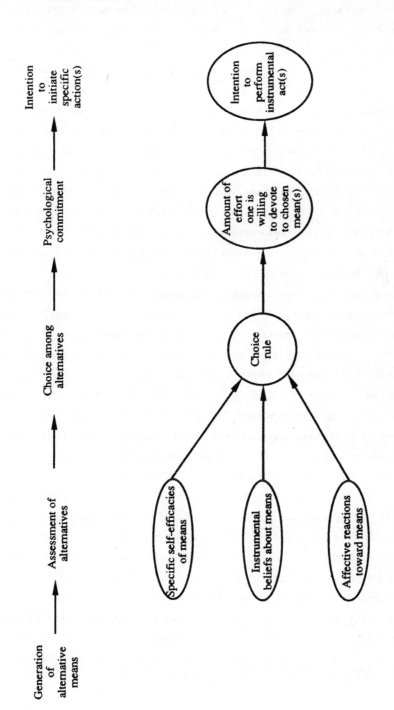

The subjective information contained in specific self-efficacy, instrumentality, and affective responses toward the possible means for goal attainment must be integrated, evaluated, and compared. This occurs through choice processes, and one or more means are then chosen according to an explicit or implicit decision rule. We will postpone discussion of the underlying choice processes until the next section where we consider goal choice and means choice processes.

After a choice of means has been made, psychological commitment processes toward these choices take hold. Commitment is reflected in the amount of effort one is willing to devote to the single means or to each of a set of means chosen. Commitment is a function of the social expectations of significant others, the amount of investment and involvement one has in the goal and in the means, and the degree of revocability of the act. It is also determined by one's self-esteem and self-concept (e.g. the desire to avoid injury to one's self-image as a person who is thoughtful, versus reckless, or as a person who follows through on one's plans).

Volitional and choice processes among means are rather abstract psychological activities which occur largely below the level of self-awareness. They become transformed into action through the operation of intention formation processes which, in turn, are conscious activities. At least, decision makers are aware of their intentions, if not the processes behind their formation. We can think of intentions to initiate an act as wilfull states that are at an intermediate level of abstraction, somewhere between abstract, mental processes and concrete, observable actions. They thus serve as a transition from reasoned and motivated processes to overt physical action.

Heretofore, attitude researchers have limited inquiry to the attitude → intention → behaviour links and have not considered the dimensionality of attitudes nor the global self-efficacy and volitional and choice processes discussed in this paper (cf. Bagozzi, 1990d). Moreover, little research has been directed at the conditions under which intentions mediate the effect of attitudes on behaviour. Bagozzi *et al.* (1989) found that the mediation depends on both measurement issues (e.g. statistical power, reliability of intention measures, validity of intentions) and the temporal and instrumental linkages between intention formaton and actual performance of a final behaviour or achievement of a goal. The likelihood that intentions mediate the attitude-behaviour relation is enhanced when measurement error in intentions is corrected for, valid measures are used, large samples employed, and the correspondences among attitudes, intentions, and behaviour are specific with respect to action, target, context, and time. Bagozzi *et al*. (1990) found that the level of effort moderates the attitude-behaviour relation as well. When the performance of behaviour requires substantial effort, the mediating role of intentions is strong. But when little effort is required, attitudes directly influence behaviour without working through intentions. Finally, Bagozzi and Yi (1989) discovered that the degree of intention formation (i.e. how well-formed intentions are) moderates the attitude-behaviour relation. Well-formed intentions completely mediate the effects of attitudes on behaviour; ill-formed intentions lead to direct effects of attitudes on behaviour. The above research is apparently the first to address volitional processes in depth but only considers some of the variables outlines in our theory. In addition, the studies were conducted in contexts other than work and family size choices and therefore more empirical work is needed both with respect to the individual mechanisms shown in figure 3 and with regard to their integration.

7.6. Choice processes

Choices are made at two points in the purposeful behaviour theory of work and family size decisions: at the point of selecting a goal or goals from among a set of goals (assuming that a choice of goals is in fact to be made) and at the point of selecting a means to implement goal pursuit (see figure 1). We propose that choices among goals and among means begin with an internal cognitive framing (Bagozzi and Van Loo, 1990). The decision maker ascertains (explicitly or implicitly) whether he or she is faced with a single-alternative or multi-alternative problem.

A *single-alternative problem* arises when the decision maker sees his or her task as either a) deciding to pursue a single goal (or perform a single action) or not, or b) deciding to continue pursuing an ongoing goal or performing an ongoing action (or discontinue pursuit or performance) or not. For example, the first situation occurs when a person decides to have a child or not, to pursue a career or not, to use contraceptives or not, or to seek occupational consuling or not; the second situation happens when one decides whether or not to quit one's job, to stop having children, to cease the use of birth control pills, or to discontinue the search for new job opportunities.

A *multi-alternative problem* emerges when the decision maker sees his or her task as one of choosing from among options. Thus one might be contemplating whether or not to have children or career or both; whether or not to use abstinence, contraceptives, or sterilization to prevent an unwanted birth; or whether or not to use one or more preparatory and search activities to obtain a job. Single-alternative and multi-alternative choice decisions involve fundamentally different psychological processes to which we now turn.

7.6.1. Single-alternative choices

To explain single-alternative choices, we can think of the decision faced by a man or women as a) for goals: choosing to adopt or not adopt a new goal (or alternatively, making up one's mind to persevere in pursuing an ongoing goal or not); b) for actions: resolving to do or not to do something new (or alternatively, making up one's mind to continue or stop doing an ongoing behaviour).

The decisions underlying this conceptualization can be expressed through expectancy-value or subjective expected utility theory. The two classes of decisions are shown in figure 4 where, for simplicity, we have presented only the cases for single-alternative choices of *actions* or behaviours (e.g. instrumental acts). It should be noted that a similar process as that outlined in figure 4 applies to single-alternative choices of *goals*. To address goals, the question at the top of figure 4 would have to be replaced with: "Does the decision address the adoption of a new goal or the abandonment of an existing goal ?" Parallel changes in the remaining boxes in figure 4 must be made to deal with goals but are not discussed further herein.

The single-alternative choice process begins with the need to make a decision, termed antecedent conditions in figure 4. In the case of the choice among goals, this might come about because a person develops his or her own set of alternative goals based on internal desires and objectives, because one experiences outcomes with respect to actual goal achievement or the failure to achieve a goal, or because a choice is "imposed" upon one as a consequence of coercive, social, moral, or other external factors (e.g. tax policies, role models, advertisements). In the case of the choice among means to pursue a felt goal, the need to make a decision arises from affective, self-efficacy, and social forces.

Figure 4. Single-alternative choices - baseline rendition

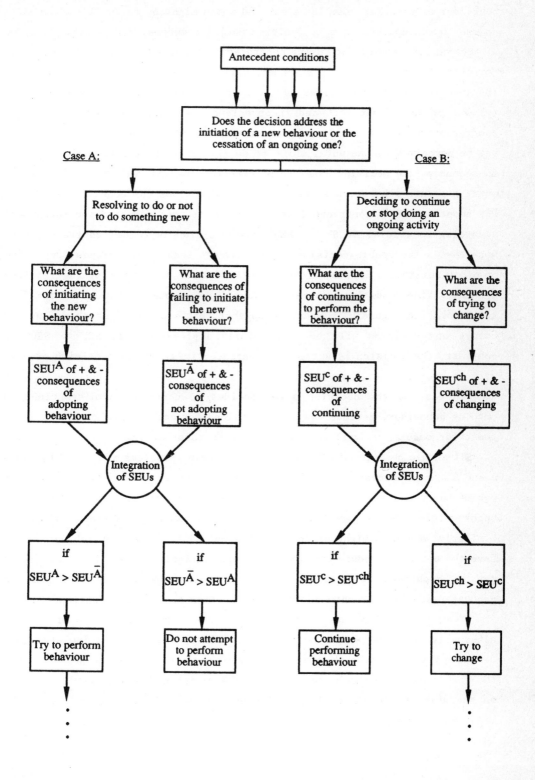

For case A in figure 4, the person faces the decision to initiate a new behaviour or not. For example, a man and woman might be faced with the choice to use contraceptives or not. Decision making commences with a consideration of the consequences of *both* using contraceptives and not using contraceptives. Moreover, either action will engender positive and negative consequences. For instance, using contraceptives may lead to more worry-free and enjoyable sex (+) but produce discomfort and inconvenience (-); whereas a failure to use contraceptives might result in greater chances of an unwanted pregnancy (-) yet be perceived as the moral thing to do (+). For each positive and negative consequence, the decision maker forms expectations and evaluations, and these enter separate subjective expected utility functions for adopting (SEU^A) and not adopting ($SEU^{\ddot{A}}$) contraceptives. The SEUs are then compared and integrated according to a rule. If $SEU^A > SEU^{\ddot{A}}$, the decision is to use contraceptives. Note that a favourable decision may or may not lead to actual use, depending on one's ability to implement the decision and the occurrence of facilitating and inhibiting conditions. Hence, we have drawn an open-ended arrow from "Try to perform" in figure 4 in order to suggest that additional steps are needed before any decision will be successfully implemented. If $SEU^{\ddot{A}} > SEU^A$ in contrast, the decision is not to use contraceptives, and the decision process will, temporarily at least, end.

In case B, the decision maker decides to continue or discontinue an ongoing behaviour. Because the steps outlined for case B in figure 4 parallel those for case A, we will not elaborate upon them herein.

It should be pointed out that decision making problems addressed by cases A and B are not necessarily all or nothing endeavours. Thus, one person might decide to enroll in a full complement of courses designed to enhance employment opportunities whereas another might decide to opt for a skeletal offering. Similarly, a person might decide not to simply quit his or her job but rather have the option to reduce employment by some variable amount. These gradients can be rephrased as single-alternative choices between nonadoption and graduated adoption or between full continuation and partial continuation.

Two additional points with respect to the conceptualization of single-alternative choices should be mentioned. First, the theory stipulates that decision makers examine the pros and cons of any alternative and act only when the former outweigh the latter. Second, the decision to act is not predicated on the absolute levels of pros and cons, per se, but rather on the levels relative to some standard used explicitly or implicitly by the decision maker.

This standard will typically encompass expectations related to one's own psychological needs and adaptation level (e.g. Helson, 1964), feeling of deprivation (e.g. Williams, 1975), and comparisons to what significant others have done or would do (e.g. Berkowitz and Walster, 1976; Suls and Miller, 1977).

A specification issue for single- as well as multi-alternative choices concerns which consequences to include in any decision. This topic will not be discussed further but is addressed in Bagozzi and Van Loo (1990).

7.6.2. Multi-alternative choices

We can think of decision making among a set of alternatives as the execution of one or more mental choice rules. As displayed in figure 5, the rules are classified as being either choice driven or simplifying. A choice driven rule is one specifying a definite policy (e.g. "choose the best alternative"). Indeed, the objective of a choice driven rule is to produce an unambiguous recommendation. A simplifying rule, in contrast, is a procedure for reducing a complex, information laden problem to a more streamlined question. No particular choice is necessarily implied, although one might be left with one or no alternatives, and therefore an implicit policy would be suggested. More often than not, however, simplifying rules do not yield an unambiguous recommendation and merely reduce the choice set. Note also that simplifying rules might be employed prior to application of choice driven rules.

There are at least two types of choice driven rules: stored processing and constructive processing rules. In *stored processing*, the decision maker treats the choice problem as a familiar one and begins by retrieving from memory attitudes (preferences) toward each alternative in a choice set. Here the individual attitudes are stored aggregates resulting from earlier assessments and integration of beliefs and evaluations performed on perceived consequences of each alternative. Following retrieval, comparisons are made across alternatives, and the best one is chosen. In *constructive processing*, the decision maker must first form an attitude toward each alternative. The expectancy-value model is one representation that might apply, but as developed elsewhere, other more complicated forms are possible as well (cf. Bagozzi, 1985). Once attitudes are formed, comparisons and choice follow in a manner similar to that noted for stored processing.

Figure 5. Types of multi-alternative choices

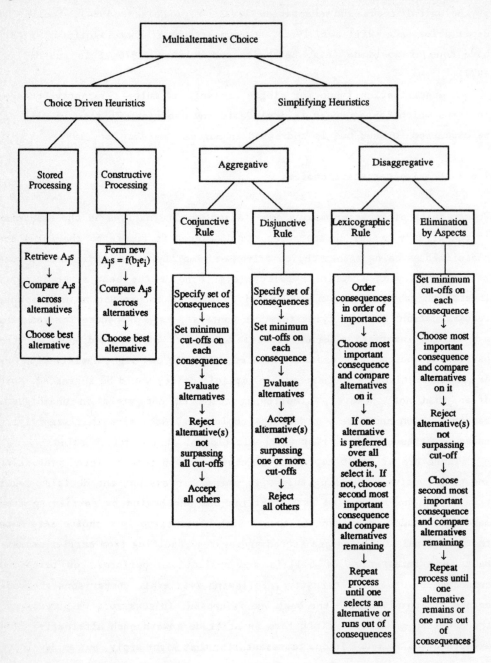

Stored and constructive processing are two classes of "processing by alternatives," i.e., comparisons are made across alternatives on the basis of aggregations of beliefs and evaluations of perceived consequences. Further, both are said to be compensatory rules because high scores on any consequence tend to make up for low scores on others.

Simplifying rules are also of two kinds: aggregative and disaggregative rules. Consider first *aggregative decision rules*. In the conjunctive rule, the decision maker begins by setting minimum cut-offs on each salient consequence. Each alternative is then evaluated on each consequence, and everyone not surpassing all cut-offs is rejected. Those scoring above all cut-offs enter the set of acceptable alternatives. In the disjunctive rule, the decision maker again sets minimum standards for each salient consequence. Alternatives are then evaluated in relation to the standard, but unlike the conjunctive rule, the disjunctive rule stipulates that acceptable alternatives need only surpass the thresholds of one or more consequences. As Wright (1974) notes, the conjunctive rule tends to weight the effects of deficiencies more heavily, whereas the disjunctive rule weights the effects of assets more heavily. As with choice driven rules, aggregative simplifying rules are applied through comparisons made at the alternative level after one has integrated information on the individual consequences for each alternative. Unlike choice driven rules, however, the aggregative simplifying rules are noncompensatory in the sense that scores above the cut-offs on one or more attributes do not atone for scores below the cut-offs on others.

Looking next at *disaggregative decision rules*, two types are noted. In the lexicographic rule, the decision maker starts by ranking consequences in order of importance. The most important consequence is then selected, and all alternatives are evaluated in relation to it. If one alternative scores higher than all others on this consequence, it is chosen. If one or more alternatives are tied on this consequence, the second most important consequence is selected, and the alternatives tied on the first are compared in relation to it. The procedure is repeated until either a superior alternative is identified or one runs out of consequences. In the elimination by aspects strategy (Tversky, 1972), the decision maker starts by setting minimum standards for each consequence. The most important consequence is selected and alternatives are compared to reject all those not surpassing the standard. If two or more alternatives remain, the second most important consequence is selected, and the remaining alternatives are compared with those falling below the standard again rejected. The procedure is repeated if necessary until either one alternative remains or one runs out of consequences. The lexicographic and elimination by aspects rules are both noncompensatory and consequence-centered in that comparisons of alternatives are done at the individual consequence level rather than at the alternative level where aggregations of consequences are first performed for each alternative. Other disaggregative decision rules are possible but will not be discussed herein.

As noted heretofore, simplifying and choice driven rules are sometimes used in tandem such that an initial stage of processing begins with an attempt to reduce the choice set down to a manageable level and then informed comparisons are made among the remaining alternatives with a well-formed rule applied. This has been termed phased strategies in the literature (e.g. Wright and Barbour, 1977). Phased strategies may be even more complex. In particular, it is hypothesized that some multi-alternative choices begin with or are preceded by a single-alternative choice or a multi-alternative choice. Thus, the decision processes outline in figure 4 can be conceived of as occurring before and interfacing with the decision processes shown in figure 5 in certain instances. Further, single-alternative decisions sometimes fall out of ongoing multi-alternative outcomes, suggesting a role for the study of the sequencing and history of choices among and between single- and multi-alternative decisions.

A considerable amount of research is now being conducted particularly with respect to multi-alternative choice contexts. It is beyond the scope of this paper to cover recent developments and the problems and opportunities with contemporary models of decision making and choice rules. For a review of the research, see Johnson and Puto (1988). Particularly pressing in our view is the need to ascertain when and why people "use" the rules they do.

7.7. Conclusion

Early research attempting to identify the psychological determinants of fertility failed miserably (e.g. Kiser and Whelpton, 1953, 1958; Westoff *et al.*, 1961), and efforts to explain career orientation as a function of psychological variables were not much more successful (e.g. Tangri, 1972). The problem with this research was the absence of a well-developed theory. Moreover, measurement techniques left much to be desired.

Beginning in the 1970s and continuing into the 1980s, researchers applied the expectancy-value model (e.g. Ajzen and Fishbein, 1980) which was based on firmer theoretical grounds than earlier approaches and employed relatively more accurate measurement techniques (e.g. Davidson and Jaccard, 1975, 1979; Sperber *et al.*, 1980; Vinokur-Kaplan, 1978). The results were measurably improved.

Nevertheless, even these investigations have limitations. In the first place, the expectancy-value model is equipped to explain behaviours, but not goals (cf. Bagozzi and Warshaw, 1990a). Secondly, the model assumes a rather simplistic form for both the integration of beliefs and evaluations and the structure of attitudes. It does not, for example, accommodate multidimensional expectancy-value representations, nor does it permit complex attitudes such as A_s, A_f, and A_p and patterns of affective responses within these. Thirdly, the role of generalized self-efficacy responses are not considered in the expectancy-value model. Fourthly, the expectancy-value model says little about volitional processes (Bagozzi, 1990d). These are represented simply as intentions. Specific self-efficacy, instrumentalities, and affective responses towards means are neglected, as are one's commitments to means. Fifthly, no provision for explaining choices are contained within the expectancy-value model. Rather, the approach applies only to a single behaviour.

The purposeful behaviour theory we developed herein builds upon the expectancy-value model yet goes well beyond it in form and substance. Significantly, the approach is grounded in sound psychological theories. To date, although a number of components and subprocesses of the purposeful behaviour theory have been tested, this has not occurred in work and family size contexts. Moreover, the entire theory has yet to be studied empirically. Future research will hopefully focus on operationalization of the approach in real world settings.

Part III
Restrictions

A BIOGRAPHIC/DEMOGRAPHIC ANALYSIS OF THE RELATIONSHIP BETWEEN FERTILITY AND OCCUPATIONAL ACTIVITY FOR WOMEN AND MARRIED COUPLES[2]

Herwig Birg
Universität Bielefeld
Institut für Bevölkerungsforschung und Sozialpolitik
Postfach 8640
4800 BIELEFELD 1
Germany

8.1. Introduction and outline

In this paper the analytical tools of the biographic theory of fertility are applied to the analysis of interdependencies of life course events which are usually treated seperately by sociologists on the one hand and economists on the other hand.

First it will be shown that the relation between decisions concerning fertility and decisions concerning occupation describes a dynamic decision process (section 2). The general characteristics of dynamic decision processes will be elaborated. Section 3 outlines the main theoretical elements of the biographic approach. Following a general introduction (section 3.1) the terminology (section 3.2) and central hypotheses of the biographic approach (section 3.3) will be described. In section 3.4 the interaction between the man's and woman's biography is analysed. Section 4 contains the empirical results obtained from a biographic survey. Finally, the main conclusions of the theoretical and empirical part are outlined in section 5.

---

[2] This paper is based on the theoretical concepts used in the research project "Labour Market Dynamics and Reproductive Behaviour" which I am directing since 1984 and which was funded by the German Research Society. The "biographic approach" propounded here arose out of this project within the framework of which a survey of 1,576 biographies was made and the theory applied. The results presented in this paper are confined to those which serve to illustrate the main parts of the theory. A full report on the empirical results will be published by my colleagues and myself in the near future. Thus, although solely responsible for the theoretical content of this paper, I would like to take this opportunity of thanking E.-J. Flöthmann and I. Reiter for their empirical work, in particular for that included here.

8.2. Dynamic decision processes

All the contributions to this book have a theoretical starting-point in common, namely that of a "preference-restrictions-behaviour scheme". This scheme implies two basic assumptions. The first of these is that there exist clear situations between which an individual can choose. For example, a woman can choose between having a paid occupation or being a housewife. The second is that the individual has certain preferences with respect to the given situations. The theoretical basis of the "preference-restrictions-behaviour scheme" therefore obviously relies on the fundamental prerequisite that restrictions and preferences can be clearly distinguished from each other. Even if it is recognized that restrictions and preferences can change in the course of time, the prerequisite that everything that belongs to the concept of "behaviour" can be uniquely separated into preferences on the one hand and restrictions on the other still has to hold good.

But is it always possible to realize such a separation? When a woman marries and then has a child this could be interpreted in the sense that the marriage and the financial security provided by the husband's income are restrictions, or boundary conditions, which, once satisfied, allow the woman to realize her preference for a child. But it could also be that the woman has chosen her husband from among a number of possible candidates so that her "restriction", namely that of wanting to have a child, is automatically satisfied in that the future husband is in full agreement. The question of what is a restriction and what a preference is hardly possible to answer for the observer. Even if the person concerned is carefully interviewed, the question is still difficult to answer, since it is perfectly possible that the woman herself doesn't know exactly.

Another everyday example serves to emphasize how difficult the problem posed generally is. When planning a holiday abroad for which the country is not definitely fixed, it is clear that a choice has to be made. Let us say that there is a preference for Spain but that other countries could also come into question. A travel catalogue is obtained in which a whole range of possibilities is presented. The catalogue has perhaps 100 pages and let us suppose that in order to find the place where the holidays in Spain begin the catalogue has to be opened somewhere and leafed through, either forwards or backwards after looking in the index. It can now happen that on the first page opened a most interesting holiday in place X is presented, interesting enough that this possibility is thoroughly read about before proceeding to look further for Spain. It can also happen that the holiday advertised is so interesting that the original preferences change and Spain is forgotten about completely. This process can be interpreted as follows: the restriction of having to search through the catalogue for Spain is transformed into the objective; the original objective, namely "Spain", was simply a step in defining a new objective so that, effectively, the old objective had the function of a boundary condition, or restriction. This exchange of objective (preference) and restriction will be called here the *"objective-restriction inversion"*.

Objective-restriction inversions occur frequently in dynamic decision processes. But two further complications arise when applying preference-restrictions-behaviour schemes to dynamic decision processes. The first of these is that of the learning capacity of human beings, who later have views and acquire opinions that they never even thought of earlier. For instance, if a woman learns, or suddenly realizes, that having children and a profession or occupation do not necessarily contradict each other in attaining her objectives of, for instance, self-realization, widening personal horizons or of making an investment for the future -objectives which were previously thought to be only attainable on the basis of a profession or occupation- then both children and an occupation suddenly appear to be means of attaining the same goal. It is then possible that children are produced to attain objectives which previously were thought to be best attainable with a profession. This process will be called *attainment-means conversion*.

The second complication lies in the simple fact that the very order of previous decision relevant phases or events in life is important in later dynamic decision making processes. Let it be supposed that a decision process is preceded by phases L and E where L is the phase of professional or occupational training in some form and E is a phase of exercising an occupation. Then the sequence (L, E) in general involves a different set of restrictions (R) for future decisions than the sequence (E, L). Schematically:

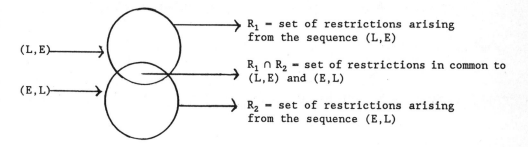

(L,E) ⟶

(E,L) ⟶

R_1 = set of restrictions arising from the sequence (L,E)

$R_1 \cap R_2$ = set of restrictions in common to (L,E) and (E,L)

R_2 = set of restrictions arising from the sequence (E,L)

Additional events can occur which have such a strong effect on the sets of
restrictions that the intersection $R_1 \cap R_2$ is empty. Such events will be called
key events (K). Schematically:

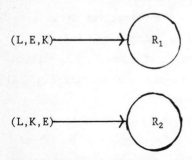

Even when, as illustrated, the phases L and E occur in the same order, a
differently interposed key event K can lead to restriction sets without any
common element. Having a child, passing final (occupational or professional)
examinations, finding a new, or separating from a previous, loved one
frequently act as key events. Different sequences do not only have effects on
the restriction sets arising but also affect the *creation of preferences*. The
above schematic description is equally well applicable to the preferences as
well as to the restrictions occurring in the course of the process.

Summarizing all the above, two levels can be distinguished in a dynamic
decision process. The preferences and restrictions belong to level 1 and the
actual decisions resulting from them can be said to belong to a level 2. The
decisions arising out of a situation i influence the restrictions and
preferences prevailing in a following decision situation i+1 (and possibly also
influence the preferences and restrictions relevant for even later situations
i+2, ...). The decisions (D_i, D_{i+1}, ...) that can be registered by an observer
in various situations and the restrictions (R_i, R_{i+1}, ...) and preferences
(P_i, P_{i+1}, ...) belonging to the psychological world of the subject, together
with exogeneous factors (X_i, X_{i+1}, ...) outside the control of the individual,
form a process which can be schematically illustrated as follows:

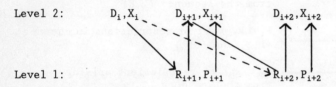

The decision sequence illustrated can be either long or short. When the sequence is long, or when the decision D_i has effects not only on the restrictions and preferences relevant for the next situation i+1 but also on those relevant for later situations, the nomenclature *long-term commitment* will be used instead of "decision" or "choice". Since long-term commitments in general determine the directions of whole processes the expression *biographic commitment* will also be used synonymously. The concept of "biographic commitment" includes both sides of the preference-restrictions-behaviour scheme, namely the subjective side to which preferences belong and the objective side to which can be counted the restrictions involved. Nearly all important decisions in life have a moral dimension. The concept of "biographic commitment" includes not only economic (financial) commitment but also moral commitment. Moral commitments always have long-term effects. But there is a significant difference between the long-term effects of moral commitments and the long-term effects of economic commitments. Economic commitments are usually only practically irreversible, in principle they are reversible. Moral commitments, however, are *irreversible in principle* - thus the term "commitment" is particularly suitable for moral decisions.

Choice of profession or occupation, of long-term partner, decisions for or against having a child, choice of place of residence and of work are all typical long-term commitments in life. These various types of commitment will be allocated to different decision levels. To do this the level 2 of the previous scheme is split up into sublevels. The intertemporal sequences described can now occur at each sublevel but can be complicated by interactions between the sublevels. When a certain decision influences decisions at other sublevels a *hierarchical decision process* is said to occur. A good example of this is the choice of profession which is usually made when quite young. This decision influences the choice of location of employment and the location of employment influences the choice of place of residence. The biographical survey to be described in the section 4 was designed for the identification and analysis of hierachical decision processes. The survey shows clear evidence of the *existence of hierarchical interval structures*.

In the extended scheme, the various decision levels can be so arranged that the number of long-term commitments decreases from top to bottom. Thus at the lowest level it can be supposed that the fewest decisions involving particularly persistent and irreversible commitments are made. Without discussing the complicated cause and effect patterns arising between the decision levels in detail, the following conceptual differentiation between decision levels can still be postulated: if decisions are made at level (i) on the basis of decisions made at the lower levels (1, 2, ..., i-1) then the decision process is said to be *statically dominated*. On the other hand, if decisions at the level (i) depend on decisions at the higher levels (i+1, i+2, ...) then the process is said to be *dynamically dominated*.

Looking at the entire decision pattern, it is difficult to identify all the relevant restrictions applying to a particular decision at a particular level, e.g. to having the second child. It is even more difficult to separate restrictions from preferences. But even if it would be possible to identify and separate all relevant restrictions and preferences, the problems of objective-restriction inversion and attainment-means conversion would still have to be solved before the topic of this paper, the relationship between fertility and the labour market behaviour of women, could be analysed on the basis of a preference-restrictions-behaviour scheme. If restrictions can replace preferences and vice versa, the theoretical basis of such a scheme becomes somewhat doubtful. However, such a pessimistic view is luckily not always justifiable. The preference-restrictions-behaviour scheme stands in doubt because decisions are regarded as being dynamic, but regarding decisions as dynamic processes itself provides a means of retaining the usefulness of the scheme. The solution is simple. It is based on the fact that the various elements of the decision process, whether or not they are interpreted as restrictions or preferences, must build a certain temporal *sequence*. Once the decision is made with which a sequence starts, the sequence cannot begin with any other element, i.e. the commitment is *irreversible*. It can be assumed that the first decision influences all that follow. The same argument can be made for the second element of the sequence, except that the second element cannot influence the first. Every human being obviously must not only express preferences in life about the things he wants to achieve but must additionally build preferences on the *order* of achievement desired. The biographic approach can be said to be a method of applying the basic principles of the preference-restrictions-behaviour scheme to the problem of biographic *sequences*.

8.3. A biographic approach

8.3.1. General introduction

The term "biography" is used in the following in both a wide and in a narrow sense. Which sense is always clear in its context. However, "biography" in its widest sense is synonymous with "story of life" which has three elements: firstly, the *experience* of the individual as part of his *inner world* which cannot be directly observed from outside; secondly, the history of the events and situations in the life of the individual which are obviously observable, and, thirdly, the history of opportunities in the individual life. The history of opportunities comprises those paths which were possible at various times but which were not realized.

The survey work performed concerns principally those elements of a biography which can be identified by means of a scientifically designed and conducted interview. These elements include the history of events and situations but also the sense of values, the attitudes, preferences and objectives of the individual. Most social scientists believe that external observation of the accessible aspects of a biography is a far too narrow view and that the more important aspects can only be determined by means of methods of hermeneutical interpretation. However, criticism of the quantitative methods mostly overlooks the fact that communication is always based on the interpretation and conversion of observable "signs" to only indirectly observable facts and implications. Writing is such a system of signs with which the most complicated phenomena of inner life can be communicated. Another system is that the simple symbols for notes on the basis of which the incredible world of music can be communicated. Both of these systems rely on an easily understandable but effective principle of communication. Everything that is communicated, however complicated, is based on the sequencing of a limited number of symbols. The biographic approach is analogous - biographies, however complicated, are comprised of ordered sets or sequences of a limited number of basic constitutive elements.

A biography therefore is not the simple sum of its constitutive elements, the sequence of the elements expresses much more. The objective of a biographic approach is to try to extract the hidden implications and content of the sequences. The following terminology should serve to develop a key with the aid of which the "language" of biographic sequences can be read.

8.3.2. Some terminology

Biographic elements
Biographic elements comprise, firstly, the various more or less temporally *extensive phases* in life which can be delineated by some means and, secondly, the *events* which occur at given points in time. Examples of phases are those of the various stages of human development (childhood, puberty, maturity, old age), the states of economic standing in life (education, active occupation, retirement) and those role sequences differentiated by sociologists such as child, teenager, marriage partner, mother or father, grandmother or grand-father, spinster or bachelor, etc. Examples of events are the successful completion of schooling (or breaking-off schooling) of various types, changes in occupation, changing residential location, acquiring permanent personal relationships (marriage), divorces, becoming a mother or father, etc. The defintition of what a biographic element is therefore appears to be somewhat open. Indeed, the definition has to be orientated on the analytical job at hand. To a large extent, however, society defines the elements through its institutional and legal structure, social norms, codes of accepted behaviour, common ethical beliefs, etc. As an example, the implications of a marriage do not depend solely on the marriage partners but are, in some areas, largely determined by the society. The social definition (and production) of biographic elements is of great importance for the application of a preference-restric-tions-behaviour scheme: *we select alternatives but we don't normally choose the alternatives that are available for selection.*

Biographic sequence and biographic universe
A biographic sequence is a listing of the constitutive events, situations and phases in the life of an individual ordered according to their time of occurrence. The biographic universe is the set of all biographic sequences that can be constructed by *permutation, variation or combination* from a given set of biographic elements with or without repetition of the elements. With only two elements, 1 and 2, the biographic universe constructed by permutation without repetition consists of just two sequences (1,2) and (2,1). Three elements provide a universe with six sequences (1,2,3), (1,3,2), (2,1,3), (2,3,1,), (3,1,2) and (3,2,1). Four elements lead to a universe with 4! = 24 sequences, five elements to one with 5! = 120 and six give a universe with 6! = 720 sequences. With only 10 elements the universe contains 3.6 million

different sequences. The use of the expression universe is intended to convey the multiplicity and astronomical size of the number of possible sequences. The biographic universe is a theoretical construction used only for analytic purposes.

Virtual biography

The virtual biography is a subset of the biographic universe. The virtual biography consists of those sequences which come, or have come, into consideration in the build-up of the factual biography of an individual. Every individual has certain preconceptions of the biographic sequences he may want to follow, of those which are possible and of those which - after certain commitments have been made - are no longer possible. All these preconceptions can affect biographical decisions, even if they are based on false arguments, inadequate information or errors of judgement. In the same way that every individual has his personal "inner world" he also has his own virtual biography. The virtual biography therefore changes with time through experience, gains in knowledge and understanding as well as by means of external influences. The factual biography is only one of the many elements of the virtual biography and perhaps is not the most important one at that.

Risk involved in long-term commitments

Every decision on the order of the biographic elements implies an irreversible commitment. Because of this irreversibility commitments contain an element of risk. Marriages, partnerships, changes of job, having children, are commitments with far-reaching consequences for the whole biography which are difficult to estimate. The less orientation there is on standardized patterns of life and the more the individual wants to "go his own way" - bearing the negative consequences if necessary -, the more consciousness there will be of the risk associated with long-term commitments. The generally increasing awareness of this risk is leading to an increasing reluctance to make long-term commitments. Marriage and having children are long-term commitments par excellence. These are being delayed or avoided altogether, and occupational commitments are being preferred which cannot be really avoided anyway in modern societies.

The risk associated with long-term commitments can be theoretically defined and numerically calculated for any virtual biography whose sequences comprise permutations of a given n biographic elements. Consider, for example, a virtual biography of which 720 sequences are comprised of six biographic elements. The factual biography arises from six commitments. With each commitment (except the last) a number of possible sequences are (implicitly or explicitly) rejected:

Commitment   Number of sequences rejected
              by the commitment:

  1               $600 = 5 * 5!$
  2                $96 = 4 * 4!$
  3                $18 = 3 * 3!$
  4                 $4 = 2 * 2!$
  5                 $1 = 1 * 1!$
  6                 $0 = 0 * 0!$
                     ———
                    719

From the 720 initial possible sequences, 719 are successively rejected by the commitments made, leaving only one, namely the factual biography. If the risk of a long-term commitment is defined as the quotient q of the number of sequences rejected by the commitment i to the total number of sequences still available at the time of commitment, then:

$$q(i,n) = \frac{(n-i)(n-i)!}{(n-i+1)!} = \frac{n-i}{n-i+1} \tag{1}$$

The risk thus associated with the first commitment in the above example is $600/720 = 0.833$ and with the second is $96/120 = 0.800$. The risk decreases with successive commitments, at the beginning of the biography it is much larger than in later phases. In investigating the historical long-term decrease in fertility rates it is important to realize that the risk of commitment increases with increasing n. The larger the number of different opportunities in life grew through industrialization, urbanization and the growth in tertiary activities as well as due to the decreasing influence of religious and social restrictions, the larger the number of biographic degrees of freedom became, with the result that the risk associated with long-term commitments also increased. The decrease in fertility was an immanent consequence of this historical process.

Biographic age

The biographic approach provides an opportunity to redefine the concept of age which is central to demography and which, until now, has usually been measured in terms of calendar time. *Biographic age* is a theoretical concept which expresses the experience gained by making biographic commitments. Experience gained is much more important for the explanation of fertility, of readiness to marry, mobility and all other relevant demographic behaviour than simply the passing of time. If the biographic age A^* of an individual is defined as the cumulative number of sequences in his virtual biography that have been effectively rejected because of the biographic commitments already made, then:

$$A^*(i,n) = \sum_{j=1}^{i} (n-j)(n-j)! = n! - (n-i)! \tag{2}$$

The individual's virtual biography comprises all the permutative sequences of n biographic elements, where i is the number of commitments made.

The biographic age in the phase i (the phase occurring after i commitments) is highly dependent on n, the number of biographic elements. In the biographic sense one is old when one has made a lot of commitments and has no (or few) alternatives left. Of course, this can happen at a young age in terms of years. On the other hand, people who live in communities or regions which are backward with respect to the general level of development, age more slowly in the biographic sense than those who live in prosperous areas where the variety and number of opportunities for different paths in life is much larger (Birg, 1987, pp. 85 and 95). On this basis the well known differentials in regional fertility can be interpreted and explained (Birg *et al.*, 1990).

Biographic divergence

The actual biography of an individual seldom coincides with his wishes. The difference between the actual and the desired sequence is called *biographic divergence* (d) or *separation*. For a virtual biography made up of the set of all permutational sequences of n biographic elements, the divergence or separation between any two of the sequences is defined as the number of phases that must be traced back from their respective ends until the two sequences become the same (Birg, 1987, p. 78).

Biographic opportunity costs

The concept of "biographic opportunity costs" is used analogously to that of economic opportunity costs. If a given commitment rules certain sequences out of the virtual biography, this implies that certain degrees of freedom have been lost and certain styles of life are no longer possible. The possibilities lost are termed the biographic opportunity costs of the commitment. Biographic opportunity costs include the economic, but not vice versa.

8.3.3. Central hypotheses of the biographic approach

With the expressions and concepts now defined it is possible to present the basic substantive hypotheses of the biographic approach. Let U be the set of sequences of the biographic universe, V the set of sequences of the virtual biography and X = U - V the set of sequences that is in the universe but not in the virtual biography. Let u, v and x be the number of sequences that are elements of the correspondingly labelled sets; u = v + x. The probability (p) of a long-term commitment in the phase i of a virtual biography with v sequences is a function of i, v and d and therefore of u, x and d:

$$p(i,v) = p_i(u,x,d) \tag{3}$$

In terms of this equation the following three hypotheses can be formulated.

Hypothesis 1
The more sequences that are contained in the biographic universe U and/or in the virtual biography V, the greater is the risk to be associated with long-term commitments and so - *ceteris paribus* - the smaller is the probability p of long-term commitment:

$$\frac{\Delta p}{\Delta u} < 0 \quad , \quad \frac{\Delta p}{\Delta v} < 0 \tag{4}$$

Hypothesis 2
The greater the divergence between the actual and the desired biographic sequence the smaller is the probability (*ceteris paribus*) of long-term commitment:

$$\frac{\Delta p}{\Delta d} < 0 \tag{5}$$

Hypothesis 3

If at a decision mode the risk of biographic commitment for two different decisions is the same, then the commitment will be made for the alternative that brings the most benefit with it. This hypothesis is directly relevant for the analysis of the connection between fertility and labour market behaviour. The implication is, for example, that if a woman has the choice of ordering the three elements L = vocational training, E = working and F = family phase including bearing her first child, then she will usually place vocational training before working and working before having a family, i.e. she will choose the sequence LEF. Firstly, the benefit of training, of gaining qualifications, before working is obvious; secondly, training is much easier at a younger age than later due to the regulations of and the conditions imposed by the educational and post-educational training systems. There is also a general concensus that training should occur without too much of a gap directly after schooling. Divergence from this rule is generally disadvantegeous. The sequence LEF therefore has more benefit associated with it than the sequences FLE and FEL.

According to the above hypotheses, the probability of a long-term commitment such as marriage or having a child must show a decreasing tendency with industrialization simply because the general process of development has steadily increased the number of biographic opportunities and degrees of freedom of the individual. However, every country comprises a number of different regional entities at a given point in time and the effects of long-term commitments are likely to be different in variously structured regions in a given period of time. If in one region the labour market is better than in others, the biographic opportunity costs will be higher there and so the less likely it will be that biographical long-term commitments will be made. Thus the probabilities of marriage and births are lower in the large, prosperous centres.

Still according to the hypotheses, it is improbable that an automatic tendency towards an increasing birth rate will occur in the industrialized countries. It is more probable that birth rates will remain at their presently low levels or decrease even further, although of course, some temporary fluctuations, induced perhaps by the business cycle or by surprisingly favourable family policies and subsidies, will occur.

8.3.4. Analysis of the biographies of couples

The biographies of the man and the woman in a (married) couple are mutually interactive. Such connected biographies are called "pair biographies". The basic concepts of section 3.2 apply also to pair biographies. However, the construction of the principal hypotheses requires considerably more differentiation than those for individuals. In the following it will be shown how the biographies of a couple interact and what the consequences are for the fertility rate. The discussion is restricted to a very simple case with the following assumptions:

A1. The sequences of the biographic universes of both the man and the woman are built up of permutations of the four biographic elements:

1 = vocational, occupational or professional education;

2 = exercising an occupation;

3 = the establishment of a permanent relationship (e.g. by marriage);

4 = having the first child.

A2. The personal relationship is mutual and occurs in binding form for both at the same time.

A3. The man and the woman have the same school education (not university education) but are not necessarily of the same age.

A4. The virtual biographies are derived from the biographic universe by deleting certain sequences according to the following rules:

CI: Occupational training comes before exercising the occupation (1 before 2) and the child comes after the establishment of the relationship (3 before 4).

CII: Both training and a working phase occur before the child is born (1 and 2 before 4).

The individual biographic universes contain 4! = 24 sequences. CI eliminates 18 of these and CII a further 3. Three sequences (1,2,3,4), (1,3,2,4) and (3,1,2,4) remain open as possibilities for the individual man and woman. These biographies of the man and the woman are connected by the element no. 3, the establishment of the personal relationship. Initially there were 24*24 = 576 combinations of biographies possible but CI and CII got rid of most of them leaving, in fact, only 9 combinations. In three of these (schematically presented in table 1 in the top left) the age of the man and the woman should be approximately the same because the sequences are synchronized. In the pair biographies P(3,1) and P(3,2) the man's occupational training begins after that of the woman is completed; this implies that the man is probably younger than the woman. If this situation is unusual in the society concerned, the number of feasible pair biographies is reduced to seven.

The further analysis is not restricted to these nine (or seven) cases but is extended firstly by omitting the element 2 (the working phase), then the element 1 (occupational training) and finally both. Table 1 therefore presents in total 64 possible pairs of sequences. The following resulting comments can be made:

(I) Although the biography matrix of table 1 is symmetrical with respect to the man and the woman, not all the symmetrical elements of the matrix are equally probable. As already mentioned, those pair biographies in which the man is younger than the woman, e.g. P(3,1):

```
Man                 3  1  2  4
Woman       1  2    3  -  -  4
```

are not usual. Improbable are also those pair biographies in which the woman works while the man does the housework and looks after the child. Not quite so improbable are those cases where the woman has profession qualifications but the man not. Nevertheless, of the 64 cases presented only the 24 in the first three rows seem to be realistic in terms of numerical significance. Four of these, P(3,1), P(3,2), P(3,4) and P(3,6), imply situations in which the woman is older than the man. It can therefore be concluded that the majority of actual pair biographies - despite the multiplicity of other combinatorial possibilities - are distributed among approximately 20 realistic biographic sequence pairings.

(II) Conflicts can additionally arise between the biographic sequences of the man and the woman, for example, as in P(1,2):

```
Man        1  2   3   -  4
Woman      1  -   3   2  4
```

Table 1. Combinations of biographic sequences of men and women in a pair
biography matrix.

The biography of the woman ...

The biography of the man ...	contains all 4 elements in the order ...			does not include element 2 (working phase)		does not include element 1 (vocational training)		... not 1 and 2
	1234	**1324**	**3124**	**134**	**314**	**234**	**324**	**34**
contains all 4 elements in the order ... — 1234	P(1,1) 1234 1234	P(1,2) 123 -4 1 -324	P(1,3) 123 -4 3124	P(1,4) 1234 1 -34	P(1,5) 123 -4 314	P(1,6) 1234 234	P(1,7) 123 -4 324	P(1,8) 1234 34
1324	P(2,1) 1 -324 123 -4	P(2,2) 1324 1324	P(2,3) 132 -4 3124	P(2,4) 1324 13 -4	P(2,5) 1 324 314	P(2,6) 1324 23 -4	P(2,7) 1324 324	P(2,8) 1324 3 -4
3124	P(3,1) 3124 123 --4	P(3,2) 3124 132 -4	P(3,3) 3124 3124	P(3,4) 3124 13 -4	P(3,5) 3124 31 4	P(3,6) 3124 23 -4	P(3,7) 3124 3 -24	P(3,8) 3124 3 -4
does not include element 2 (working phase) — 134	P(4,1) 1 -34 1234	P(4,2) 13 -4 1324	P(4,3) 13 -4 3124	P(4,4) 134 134	P(4,5) 13 -4 314	P(4,6) 134 234	P(4,7) 13 -4 324	P(4,8) 134 34
314	P(5,1) 31 4 123 -4	P(5,2) 314 1324	P(5,3) 31 -4 3124	P(5,4) 314 13 -4	P(5,5) 314 314	P(5,6) 314 23 -4	P(5,7) 314 324	P(5,8) 314 3 -4
does not include element 1 (vocational training) — 234	P(6,1) 234 1234	P(6,2) 23 -4 1324	P(6,3) 23 -4 3124	P(6,4) 234 134	P(6,5) 2 3 -4 314	P(6,6) 234 234	P(6,7) 23 -4 324	P(6,8) 234 34
324	P(7,1) 324 123 -4	P(7,2) 324 1324	P(7,3) 3 -24 3124	P(7,4) 324 13 -4	P(7,5) 324 314	P(7,6) 324 23 -4	P(7,7) 324 324	P(7,8) 324 3 -4
not 1 and 2 — 34	P(8,1) 34 1234	P(8,2) 3 -4 1324	P(8,3) 3 -4 3124	P(8,4) 34 134	P(8,5) 3 -4 314	P(8,6) 34 234	P(8,7) 3 -4 324	P(8,8) 34 34

Explanation: The first row in each element of the matrix is the sequence of the man, the second is that for the woman. Definitions: 1 = vocational training, 2 = working phase, 3 = mutual permanent relationship established, 4 = birth of first child. Initially there are 24 (= 4!) sequences for the man and 24 for the woman. Of the resulting 576 pair biographies the 64 are presented here that satisfy the conditions (i) training before working (1 before 2) and permanent relationship before child (3 before 4), (ii) the child arrives after training and working (1 and 2 before 4) and (iii) the relationship occurs mutually which implies that the element 3 for man and woman must align.

It is not very likely that this pair will come together because the man enters into a binding relationship only after working and the woman before working. On the other hand, because the occupational training has taken place together the potential partners are likely to be of the same age. The two situations are therefore only compatible if the woman does absolutely nothing (in the sense of this analysis) for quite a while during which the man is working and deciding whether to enter into a permanent relationship or not. Similarily, the case $P(1,3)$:

Man	1	2	3	-	-	4
Woman			3	1	2	4

implies a situation in which the woman is much younger than the man. These examples serve to demonstrate that the *timing* of entering into a permanent personal relationship plays a *key role* in the creation of compatible and successful pair biographies and therefore finally for the fertility rate of the population.

(III) Finally, the examples demonstrate to which extent individual and pair biographies are usually restricted by quite simple considerations. Let n be the number of biographic elements that permutationally build the sequences and h be the number of elements that - due to restrictions - have to occur in a given order ($h \leq n$). The number of sequences without restrictions is n! and with restrictions it is:

$$s = \frac{n!}{h!} \tag{6}$$

If a further restriction implies that another k elements also have to have a given order, then:

$$s = \frac{n!}{h!k!} \tag{7}$$

If the sequences of the man contain m elements and those of the woman n elements and if m_1 elements for the man and n_1 elements for the woman have to occur in a given order, then the number of pair biographies becomes:

$$s_{m,n} = \frac{m!}{m_1!} * \frac{n!}{n_1!} \tag{8}$$

The reductions effected by restrictions are much more significant for pair biographies than for individual biographies. If $m = n$ and $m_1 = n_1$, then the reduction factor for the individual biographies is $1/m_1!$ but it is $1/(m_1!)^2$ for the set of pair biographies. This implies that the difficulties of planning the future are much greater for pairs when restrictions are introduced at individual level on *both sides*. The restriction that both the man and the woman should have occupational training before they work is much more difficult to fulfill at the pair level than for the separate individuals.

8.4. Application

8.4.1. A biographic survey

In order to test the biographic theory developed, a survey of 1,576 biographies was made. The sampling was random under the condition of a 50/50 composition of men and women. The survey was restricted to the cohorts of 1950 and 1955. The cohorts of 1950 entered into the labour market around 1970, i.e. into a situation of full employment when the official unemployment rate stood at a miraculous 0.8%. Those born in 1955 entered into the labour market around 1975 when, due to the oil crisis, unemployment had risen to approximately 5%. Although born only five years apart, the two groups were faced with significantly different conditions in planning their careers.

In addition, regional differences in the labour market situations of those interviewed imposed restrictions at least as strong as those generally existing between the cohorts. The survey sample was distributed over communities of three types of regions, namely over

- *regions type 1* with favourable labour market conditions (the cities of Düsseldorf and Hannover),
- *regions type 2* with unfavourable conditions (the coal and steel areas Bochum and Gelsenkirchen) and
- *regions type 3* (the rural communities of Ahaus, Vreden, Gronau and Leer).

Approximately 10% of the interviews were of couples. The single interviews also contained questions for the partner - if the randomly chosen person in fact had a permanent partnerschip.

The interview technique used will not be discussed in detail here exept to note that the standardized questionnaire was moduled to accommodate a large variety of biographies. The questionnaire was essentially job-oriented, i.e. for each place of employment a separate module (sub-questionnaire) was used with the implication that the interview for a person who had had only three jobs in life was much shorter than that for someone who had had 10 or 20. A further characteristic of the questionnaire was that the questions to the *occupational biography*, the *family biography* and the *residential biography* were not separately grouped but posed intermingled with the deliberate intention that memory in one area would refresh - if necessary - memory in the others. On average each biography produced approximately 2,000 or even more pieces of information of both quantitative and qualitative natures. Although the analysis of this data began only recently, a number of significant results have already been obtained.

8.4.2. Empirical results

Without doubt the most important result is that the principal hypothesis held good that the fertility levels of the two cohorts should be significantly different and that the regional variations are at least as important (table 2).

The question as to whether the type of the biographic sequences has the expected considerable effect on fertility and occupational behaviour is extremely important. Although empirical analysis has only just started, there

Table 2. Fertility rates cumulated up to the age of 31, by region, cohort and birth order.

	Cohort 1950				Cohort 1955			
	first born	second born	third born	total	first born	second born	third born	total
Region 1	658	336	82	1096	516	252	45	813
Region 2	740	397	75	1219	754	366	77	1204
Region 3	875	694	208	1833	786	414	171	1386
Total	734	431	104	1291	659	327	82	1074

Note: the table lists the number of births of order n per 1000 women.

seems to be strong evidence that the structure of the sequence of the
biographic elements actually does have significant effects. How varied these
sequences can be, is illustrated by the fact that the list of biographic
elements contains 30 different positions. In addition to these, the various
places of residence, the occasions of marriage and similar family events also
have to be considered. Even if only 10 of the 30 elements are considered for
building sequences, the resulting number of sequences is still almost astronomical. For the first analysis the 30 positions were therefore aggregated
to only three, namely:

L = professional/occupational/vocational training
E = phase of work
F = family phase

The period of employment E includes not only actively working but also periods
of unemployment and the phase of maternity leave. All possible forms of
occupational training were aggregated into L. How this aggregation was made
can be illustrated by an example. A married woman, born in 1950, and living
in Hannover left school at the age of 16 and then went through the following
phases:

- vocational training (apprenticeship) ——————————————— L
- obtained employment with firm of apprenticeship ———┐
- change of employer (two times) ———————————————┘ E
- housewife (without employment) ——————————————— F
- occupational activity (again) ————————————————┐
- unemployed ——————————————————————————————————┤
- another job —————————————————————————————————┤ E
- change of employer ——————————————————————————┘

This sequence was aggregated as shown, giving the sequence LEFE which was then
carried forward in the analysis. To this can be matched the sequences of places
of residence (M) and of other significant elements such as marriage and the
birth of children in order to carry out some of the more important extensions
(Birg and Flöthmann, 1990).

   The sequence given as an example above contains by definition only the
elements L, E and F. By these elements various biographic sequences can be

modeled using the mathematical techniques of permutation, variation and combination. For the following the mathematical technique of variation is adopted. For the empirical analysis two restrictions are applied: (1) Each element can occur more than once in a sequence but without following one another in position. (2) Each sequence has a maximum number of 6 elements. It can be shown that the biographic universe of this model consists of exactly 189 sequences (Birg *et al.*, 1989, pp. 9 and 24). This model serves as a theoretical basis for the interpretation of the following empirical results.

(I) Sex specific differences of biographic sequences
According to the theoretical model 189 types of sequences are possible. In reality, however, only 57 different types occur (table 3). Women show a much greater variety of types than men (table 4). Approximately 50% of women's sequences concentrate on the two types LE and LEF, whereas 60% of the men's sequences concentrate on the only type LE (tabel 4). The root LE and the following four extensions of this root made up the biographies of 67% of the women interviewed; for men this was 77%:

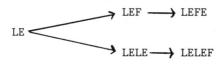

Because of the double responsibility of having to earn money and manage the home with children, women have more differentiated and more complicated biographies. The family phase occurs more frequently the longer a sequence is. For sequences with 6 phases this was 81%, with two phases 18%. When an F occurs in a woman's sequence it is nearly always in the last or next to the last position. For economically active women with children the elemtnes E and F very often occur at the same time. In the big cities (Region 1 and 2) about 50% of the women with children had the double element E/F (F combined with E), in the rural communities (region 3) the proportion was about 40%.

(II) Cohort and parity specific differences of fertility between regions
The differences in cohort and parity specific fertility rates between regions exceed more than 200% (table 2). These differences are due to the different sequence structures of the region and cohort specific biographies.

Table 3. Dendrogram of the biographic sequences of women of cohort 1950, by region.

No.	Type of Sequence	Frequency of Sequence Region 1	Region 2	Region 3	% Region 1	% Region 2	% Region 3
1	LELELE	3	3		2.1	2.1	
2	LELEL	1	2		0.7	1.4	
3	LELELF						
4	LELE	8	7		5.5	4.8	
5	LELEF	5	4	3	3.4	2.8	4.3
6	LELEFE	2	2		1.4	1.4	
7	LEL	3			2.1		
8	LELFLF						
9	LELF	2			1.4		
10	LELFE	2			1.4		
11	LE	35	25	15	24.0	17.2	21.4
12	LEFLE						
13	LEFLEF			1			1.4
14	LEFLF						
15	LEFLFE		1			0.7	
16	LEF	33	38	25	22.6	26.2	35.7
17	LEFELE						
18	LEFE	21	20	4	14.4	13.8	5.7
19	LEFEF	3	11	3	2.1	7.6	4.3
20	LEFEFE	5	9	2	3.4	6.2	2.9
21	L						
22	LFLE	2			1.4		
23	LFLEF	1			0.7		
24	LFL						
25	LFLFLE			1			1.4
26	LFLFL						
27	LF		3	2		2.1	2.9
28	LFELEL						
29	LFE	4		1	2.7		1.4
30	LFEFL						
31	LFEF						
32	LFEFE			1			1.4
33	LFEFEF			1			1.4
34	ELELE		1			0.7	
35	ELELEF			1			1.4
36	ELEL						
37	ELE	4	1	2	2.7	0.7	2.9
38	ELEF	2			1.4		
39	ELEFE	1			0.7		
40	EL						
41	ELFLE						
42	ELFL						
43	ELF						
44	ELFE						
45	E	7	1		4.8	0.7	
46	EFLFE						
47	EF	2	6	3	1.4	4.1	4.3
48	EFE		5	2		3.4	2.9
49	EFEF		1	1		0.7	1.4
50	EFEFE		2			1.4	
51	FLELEF			1			1.4
52	FLE						
53	FLFEF			1			1.4
54	FLFEFE		1			0.7	
55	F		1			0.7	
56	FEF		1			0.7	
57	FEFEF						
	Total	146	145	70	100.0	100.0	100.0

L = professional training, E = phase of work and F = family phase
About 40-50% of the elements E are combined with F. See text.

Table 4. Relative frequencies of the various types of biographic sequences
         for cohort 1950 (in %).

type of sequence	Women Cohort 1950			Men Cohort 1950		
	Region 1	Region 2	Region 3	Region 1	Region 2	Region 3
LELE	5.5	4.8	-	26.8	21.2	23.1
LELEF	3.4	2.8	4.3	-	-	-
LE	24.0	17.2	21.4	61.3	65.8	53.8
LEF	22.6	26.2	35.7	-	-	-
LEFE	14.4	13.8	5.7	-	-	-
LEFEF	2.1	7.6	4.3	-	-	-
LEFEFE	3.4	6.2	2.9	-	-	-
LFE	2.7	-	1.4	-	-	-
ELE	2.7	0.7	2.9	5.6	4.1	7.7
E	4.8	0.7	-	0.7	1.4	3.1
Others	14.4	20.0	21.4	5.6	7.5	12.3
Total	100.0	100.0	100.0	100.0	100.0	100.0

Note: About 40-50% of the elements E are combined with F, see text.

For example, in region 1 only 60% of the women's sequences of cohort 1950
beginning with LE ... contained the element F, in regions 2 and 3 this proportion was 69% and 70% respectively.

(III) Fertility and migration

A complete residential history biography is existing for each individual.
With these biographic data it is possible to subdivide the population of each
region into a native and an immigrated population. The natives are defined as
being that population which was born in a certain region and has never lived
in any other region. The data show that the regional fertility differentials
are mainly based on fertility differentials of the *native population*.
Consequently, the regional fertility differentials cannot be exclusively
attributed to migration (Birg *et al.*, 1989).

(IV) Re-entry effect

The average number of children of women who re-enter the labour market after
a family phase is approximately 30% lower than that of women (belonging to the

same cohort and region) who do not re-enter the labour market. This *re-entry effect* (r) can be calculated as follows:

$$r = \frac{\text{children per woman of sequence LEFE}}{\text{children per woman of sequence LEF}}$$

The re-entry effect is highest for women with a high level of education: Low level of education: r=0.66, medium level of education: r=0.79, high level of education: r=0.59. In addition, the re-entry effect is greater in cities with favourable labour market conditions than in rural communities: Düsseldorf (0.62), Hannover (0.67), Bochum (0.87), Gelsenkirchen (0.71), rural region 3 (0.74).

(V) Conditional birth probabilities and long-term commitments

The large regional fertility differentials support the central hypothesis of the biographic approach. The analysis of the regional nuptiality differentials gives further support (Birg *et al.*, forthcoming). The results, however, will not be illustrated here due to limited space. Support can also be drawn from the analysis of cohort and parity specific fertility rates, which are now available for all cohorts of the FRG after the Second World War (Birg *et al.*, 1990, pp. 34-37). These data enable a calculation of conditional birth probabilities. It appears that the conditional probability for a woman to have her second child is *higher* than the conditional probability for a woman without children to have her first child. Referring to the biographic theory this important fact can be interpreted as follows: More biographic alternatives are eliminated from the biographic choice set at birth of the first child than at birth of the second child. For that reason the biographic risk is bigger (and the birth probability smaller) at birth of the first child than at birth of the second child. This is the reason why an *increasing polarization of the population* can be observed in two groups with and without children.

8.5. Conclusions

Biographies can be regarded as the outcome of dynamic decision processes. In these processes preferences and restrictions can change their parts. In that case phenomena like "objective-restrictions inversion" and "attainment-means conversion" will appear. People make choices between alternatives, but they do not choose the alternatives which are available for selection. Whether a preference to have a child developes at all depends on the previous commitments in the occupational biography. On the other hand a commitment regarding the birth of a child can influence future occupational preferences. The *concept of biographic commitments* includes both sides of the preference-restrictions-behaviour scheme, namely the subjective side to which preferences belong and the objective side to which the restrictions involved can be counted. The biographic approach can be said to be a method of applying the principles of the preference-restrictions-behaviour scheme to the problem of biographic sequences.

Long-term biographic commitments are associated with a greater risk the larger the number of alternatives and options in life that is eliminated by the commitments. The bigger the risk of a commitment is, the less likely it is that it will be entered into. Industrialization and urbanization processes have multiplied the number of occupational opportunities available to everyone but in particular for women through the creation of jobs in the service sector. The decrease in the fertility rate to be observed in all countries is the most marked in the prosperous service centre cities where the majority of employment opportunities for women are to be found.

In rural areas and in regions with unfavourable labour market conditions a biographic commitment in the form of having a child implies less loss of opportunity than in areas with favourable conditions. The frequency of births is therefore higher in depressed areas than in areas of economic growth. In societies whose economic and social systems are based on the competition principle, family and occupational objectives are difficult to reconcile. The decrease in the completed fertility rate in nearly all the so-called developed countries can be traced to this inherent conflict. Economic prosperity and demographic stability - if this is defined as maintaining the present level of population - appear to be mutually exclusive as macro-economic and macro-demographic objectives in the same way that price stability, economic growth and balance of international trade are mutually exclusive. The "magic triangle" of the economists has now to include demographic effects and so be extended to a "magic polygon".

LABOUR MARKET RESTRICTIONS AND THE ROLE
OF PREFERENCES IN FAMILY ECONOMICS[1]

Klaus F. Zimmermann and John P. De New
Ludwig-Maximilians-Universität München
Seminar für Arbeits- und Bevölkerungsökonomie
Ludwigstraße 28 RG
8000 MÜNCHEN 40
Germany

9.1. Introduction

According to Becker

"The economic approach contributes important insights toward explaining the large decline in birth rates during the past 100 years, the rapid expansion in the labour force participation of married women after the 1950s, the explosive advance in divorce rates during the past two decades, and other major changes in the family. Family economics is now a respectable and growing field." (Becker, 1988, p. 3).

On the basis of this, one might be tempted to argue

"that what appear to be sociological phenomena are in fact economic phenomena thereby rendering them completely understandable in terms of pure economic concepts. On the principle of Occam's Razor this is stating that all the family's activities can be viewed, with greater ease and more insight, as problems of maximising utility subject to constraints rather than attempts to pursue the goals which are posited by sociologists." (Cameron, 1985, pp. 43-44).

We are not willing to go so far. This is justified by sufficiently strong complaints about the limitations of the maximization framework. There are useful elements for rival theories like preference formation approaches, habit formation and reference group behaviour, and concepts of bounded rationality, among others (see Leibenstein, 1957, 1980; Easterlin *et al.*, 1980; Zimmermann, 1985). "Certainly, there is a natural desire to have a theory that spares us the need to apply a rational model to behaviour concerning family size. But

---

[1] Financial support of the German Science Foundation (DFG) in the form of a project grant and a Heisenberg Fellowship to the first author is gratefully acknowledged. We wish to thank Jacques Siegers and conference participants for many useful comments.

at present we have no such a model." (Ben-Porath, 1980, p. 51). Also, we are a far cry away from incorporating those ideas fruitfully in the neoclassical model.

To stimulate discussion and to underline the power of the economic approach, we go to the extreme: we claim that consumption preferences play no sufficient role within an economic framework of labour force participation and fertility as soon as labour is demand-side rationed. We argue that this result is particularly valid in a framework that explains child costs in the context of social norms, a case that was made by Okun (1960) against Becker (1960). We think that this finding is particularly realistic in the face of obvious institutional constraints in the labour market causing all kinds of over- and under-employment, and of the increased relevance of unemployment.

Section 2 of the paper contains a brief review of the economic theory of fertility and labour force participation. Section 3 outlines a base model. Section 4 contains simulations in this framework. Section 5 concludes.

9.2. Theory of fertility and labour force participation: review

A crucial step in the development of population theory has been the endogenization of fertility. Although classical economists such as Adam Smith, Thomas Robert Malthus and David Ricardo were treating population as endogenous, this tradition was ignored when the theory of optimum population emerged as an attractive instrument to economic demographers in the first half of the 20th century (see Zimmermann, 1989a). This has only recently changed.

The achievements in this field were inspired by seminal contributions of Leibenstein (1957) and Becker (1960) who studied fertility behaviour within the framework of consumer theory. Hence the dominating model of fertility analysis today is based on a theory of rational individuals maximizing utility under given constraints. This approach is sometimes called the Chicago school model. A rival framework is the Pennsylvania school model which gives more emphasis to preference formation, supply factors and behaviour under imperfect information (e.g. Easterlin *et al.*, 1980).

However, even in the Chicago school model the traditional framework of household choices was enriched in many ways. Parents decide about the quantity and quality of their children: they care about their well-being. A household production framework allows one to incorporate various restrictions in modelling individual choices. Specifically, the time-cost of child-rearing is noted and children are considered to be more time-intensive than other home production activities. As a positive economic theory, home production must be assumed to be female time-intensive. The model therefore provides an explanation of female time allocation between work in the home and labour market work, as well as a rationale for the observed negative correlation between female labour supply and fertility. Both variables are seen as jointly endogenous to family decision making (Mincer, 1963).

A central puzzle of the analysis of population change is the observed negative correlation between fertility and economic development or income. The neoclassical theory of fertility suggests two major reasons for fertility decline. First, the *cost of time hypothesis* implies that the (relative) increase of female wages in the process of economic development is a particular relevant cause. Second, the *quantity-quality approach* to fertility choice predicts that, with rising income, there is likely to be a substitution effect from quantity to quality of children. An increase of quality per child implies an (endogenous) increase of expenditures per child and this endogenous (and negative) price effect may more than compensate the positive income effect. Hence, fertility may decline *even if* children are not inferior "goods." A precondition for this is, however, that the budget constraint is non-linear. Also, the assumption that children are time-intensive is occasionally criticized on empirical grounds (Robinson, 1987).

An alternative explanation for the negative correlation between fertility and income within the neoclassical framework was recently developed by Zimmermann (1987, 1989a, 1989b). It is argued that an increase in the *variety of goods* available to the consumers contribute to the *long-run factors* explaining fertility decline. This extends an idea presented by the German economist Lujo Brentano (1909, 1910). It is also worthy to note that Brentano had already fully outlined all central elements of modern family economics. Though this contribution was never completely forgotten in German demography (see Zimmermann, 1988, 1989a, 1989b) it seems to be time to remember this old German tradition.

Although Leibenstein (1957) and Becker (1960) clearly used a cost-benefit approach to analyse fertility decisions, economics of the family had some way to go until the basic elements outlined were developed. This stage was reached with the publication of the Chicago conference volume edited by Schultz (1974). Becker (1960) applied the standard theory to the family treating children as consumer "durables." At a time when fertility was again rising in the United States, he supported the Malthusian view of a positive relationship between income and fertility. "Malthus' famous discussion was built upon a strongly economic framework; mine can be viewed as a generalization and development of his." (Becker, 1960, p. 209). He introduced the new element "quality" of children, but concluded (p. 217) that theory suggests "that a rise in income would increase both the quality and quantity of children desired." This result was based on the assumption that children are not inferior goods. Different empirical correlations were explained by "general evidence that contraceptive knowledge has been positively related to income. ... Such evidence does little more than suggest that differential knowledge of contraceptive techniques might explain the negative relationship between fertility and income." (Becker, 1960, p. 218).

The persistence of a negative income effect in later empirical studies and an ongoing discussion about this problem inspired the ingenious paper by Becker and Lewis (1974). It demonstrates that given a certain non-linear interaction of costs for quantity and quality of children, an endogenous price effect may drive the observed income elasticities to be negative, though the linear (or "true") income effect is positive. The basic idea can be traced to Becker (1960); especially to footnote 10 on page 215; however, this was not yet sufficiently developed. Also, the other central element of modern family economics, the time cost of rearing children, was later introduced by Mincer (1963). A general theory of home production was provided by Becker (1965), Lancaster (1966) and Muth (1966), and this theory is related to earlier contributions by Mitchell (1912) and Reid (1934). However, the basic elements of home production which are crucial for fertility decisions are implicitly contained in the Mincer (1963) study.

Brentano (1909) - Brentano (1910) is a poor summary of the brilliantly written German book - already contains all key elements of the modern economic theory of the family: rational choice of utility maximizing individuals, time costs of rearing children, substitution of quantity by quality of children. Instead of "quality", Brentano used the term "refinement in the love of children", and he defines it in exactly the same way as Beckér his concept of quality. The theory was already outlined in a series of newspaper articles in a public debate of Brentano with the German economist Adolph Wagner in 1901 (see Zimmermann, 1988, for a detailed discussion of this issue), in which Brentano took the position that an increase in income causes a fertility decline. Actually, the debate was life-long, originating in 1871 when Brentano completed his "Habilitation with Wagner" in Berlin. His critical evaluation of the wage fund theory of Malthus was closely related to the population issue (see Brentano, 1872, pp. 170-186). The crucial point of his critique was that increasing prosperity would be linked with declining fertility. It is useful noting that fertility decline in Germany was only modest until 1900, but became drastic between 1901 and the first world war. Mombert (1907), a former student of Brentano, published a rich empirical study confirming Brentano's position and Brentano (1909) contains additional statistical material. In 1909, Brentano's aim was to defeat the whole Malthusian theory. In that, his motive was quite different from Becker's in 1960.

Beyond the modern analysis of fertility, Brentano (1909), emphasizes the concept of *variety of goods*. There are two aspects: (a) aith increasing variety of goods, the utility maximization principle becomes more relevant for individual decisions; (b) an increase of the variety of goods induces a pressure to substitute consumption goods for children. The validity of the second hypothesis was confirmed in a neoclassical framework by Zimmermann (1987, 1989a, 1989b).

Easterlin (1987) is the major reference for an economic model of lifetime fertility in which preference formation plays a major role. This approach proposes that consumption experiences during adolescence determine the weights individuals place on material goods as sources of satisfaction. Individuals from high-income families, therefore, have built up strong preferences for material goods which will influence their fertility decisions.

In what follows, we will only indirectly evaluate the Easterlin theory. We strip down the economic framework to the basics. First, the elements are explained. Second, some simulations explore the potentials to mimic observed factual behaviour.

9.3. The framework with restricted and unrestricted labour

An elementary lifetime model is discussed which exhibits the basic propositions of modern family economics. A modification of a framework suggested by Zimmermann (1985, 1986) is used. A representative household is studied. A family consists of one parent and her kids. Utility is derived from the fertility rate K and from a consumption good or consumption bundle C. However,

the central findings of family economics can be obtained by an investigation
of family *constraints* alone.

All that is necessary are two definitions and some simple assumptions
about the home production technology:

$$1 = H + L \; ; \; 0 < H , L < 1 \tag{1}$$

$$C + PX = WL + M \tag{2}$$

$$H = \alpha C + \beta K \; ; \; 0 \le \alpha, \beta < 1 \tag{3}$$

$$X/K = \gamma C \; ; \; 0 < \gamma < 1 \tag{4}$$

Equation (1) is the time constraint of the parent: she works at home (H) or
in the market (L), and total time available is normalized to 1. Equation (2)
is the family budget constraint deflated by the price index of consumption:
WL + M is real family income, W is the real wage rate and M is a real initial
endowment (wealth). P is the relative price of goods devoted to children, and
C and X are market goods consumed by the parent and the kids, respectively.

Equations (3)-(4) represent home production technology. Equation (3)
defines the time spent on work in the home by the parent; αC is her time spent
on consumption, βK the necessary time to rear children, and α and β are
parameters. Equation (4) assumes a proportional relationship between consumption per kid X/K and consumption by the parent. It is assumed that a social
norm forces her to provide each child with a similar quality of life that she
herself enjoys.

Note that equations (1)-(4) imply the full budget constraint

$$C(1 + \alpha W) + K(P\gamma C + W\beta) = W + M = Y \tag{5}$$

where Y stands for potential income. The related graph to equation (5) is
given by figure 1, e.g. AEB, with A = (W + M)/(1 + αW) and B = (W + M)/Wβ.
Assume wealth M to be proportional to the real wage rate W. An increase of the
real wage rate W leaves B unchanged, whereas A moves up to D. A rise of P, the
relative price of goods consumed by kids, increases the curvature of the budget
line. The first effect implies a shift of the curve from AEB to DB, the second

a shift to AFB. Both mechanisms discriminate against family size during the process of long-run economic expansion.

Figure 1. Family C-K restrictions with unrationed labour

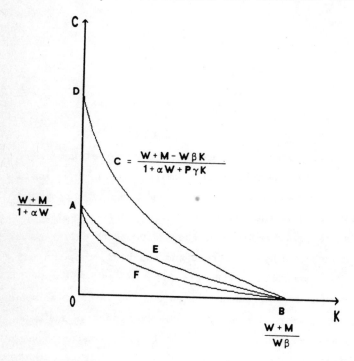

In most empirically relevant situations, labour market work is subject to demand-side constraints, either because of institutional restrictions or involuntary unemployment. In this case,

$$1 = H + \bar{L} \; ; \; 0 < H, \bar{L} < 1, \tag{1a}$$

in which we ignore the possibility of $\bar{L}=0$ for lifetime labour supply. From (1a) and (3), it follows that

$$(1 - \bar{L}) = \alpha C + \beta K \; , \; \text{or} \tag{6}$$

$$C = [\, (1 - \bar{L}) - \beta K \,] \, / \, \alpha. \tag{6a}$$

From (1a), (2) and (4), we obtain

$$C(1 + P\gamma K) = \overline{W}\overline{L} + M \text{ , or} \tag{7}$$

$$C = \frac{\overline{W}\overline{L} + M}{1 + P\gamma K}. \tag{7a}$$

For $(1 - \overline{L})/\alpha > \overline{W}\overline{L} + M$, there is a *unique* solution. (For $\alpha=0.0$, this is auto-matically the case.) This situation is illustrated in figure 2 with equilibrium at point E. For $(1 - \overline{L})/\alpha < \overline{W}\overline{L} + M$, there is likely either *no* solution, or, failing that, there are *two* solutions. In the simulations in section 4, we will assume $(1 - \overline{L})/\alpha > \overline{W}\overline{L} + M$.

Figure 2 illustrates clearly that there is only one solution in the (C,K)-space, viz. E. *Preferences play no role* in the determination of this combination, though a utility index function will pass through this point. It is easy to see how economic factors affect individual behaviour: an increase of L will shift the line AB to the left, pushing D upwards; both effects result in a decline of fertility K and an increase of market goods consumed by the parent C. Hence, a reduction of work possibilities in the labour market will

Figure 2. Family C-K restrictions with rationed labour

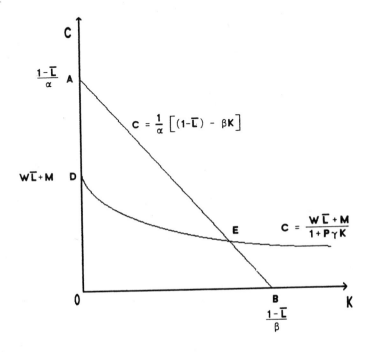

increase child-birth. The same result holds for larger α's, the parameter reflecting time spent per unit of consumption in the household, and smaller β's, the parameter measuring the time spent per kid. An increase of the wage real rate W or wealth M will shift the D-curve upwards and reduce fertility and stimulate consumption. An increase of the relative price P strengthens the curvature of the D-curve and *increases* fertility and decreases consumption.

This discussion demonstrates that it is possible to obtain a wide range of interesting results based on the restrictions alone. Nevertheless, we use a utility index function which is essential in obtaining clear findings in the unrationed case. A very simple version is the Stone-Geary utility function

$$\log U = \mu \, \log C + (1 - \mu) \, \log K, \quad 0 < \mu < 1, \tag{8}$$

which excludes inferior activities, if the constraint is linear. However, maximization of the utility function (8) with respect to the non-linear constraint (5) yields a potential negative income effect on fertility: In the *unrationed case*, $\partial K / \partial M < 0$ if

$$\frac{\mu}{1 - \mu} > 1 + \frac{1 + \alpha W}{P \gamma K}. \tag{9}$$

For a more general discussion of such a model see Zimmermann (1985).

The traditional Becker-model of the family allows average resources spent on kids, $Q = X/K$, to enter the utility function directly. This would modify (8) to

$$\log U = \mu_1 \, \log C + \mu_2 \, \log K + \mu_3 \, \log Q, \quad \mu_1, \, \mu_2, \, \mu_3 > 0, \tag{8a}$$

and $\mu_1 + \mu_2 + \mu_3 = 1$. However, replacing Q by use of (4) yields:

$$\log U = (\mu_1 + \mu_3) \, \log C + \mu_2 \, \log K + \mu_3 \, \log \gamma . \tag{8b}$$

Hence, (8b) is behaviourally equivalent to (8).

It is easy to derive the comparative statics of the rationed and unrationed models, but in order to avoid an overly technical presentation, and to explore the sensivity of the results to various parameter values more carefully, we have carried out a simulation study, which will be explained in the next section.

9.4. A simulation study

There are many ways of exploring the richness of the model. We have discussed two distinct versions, the restricted and the unrestricted case. In modelling changes, one has to define starting values. Should they be chosen randomly, or should they be linked to the case under study, e.g. come from the optimization procedure itself ? We decided in favour of starting values that are consistent with an optimization program.

There are four parameters: α, β reflecting "home-production technology", γ representing social norms, and μ individual preferences; furthermore, initial levels of wealth M, real wage rate W and relative price of goods devoted to children P have to be given. After the choice of a respective space, the labour rationed or unrationed optimal values of consumption and fertility can be calculated. In the unrationed case, these results follow from the utility maximization program. Here, also an optimal labour supply can be calculated. Given these optima or starting values, we ask: what are the implications for consumption, fertility and labour, if changes in the exogenous variables (i) price of kid's resources, (ii) price effect of wage, (iii) non-labour income are considered, and individuals are *now* (a) unrationed or (b) rationed in the labour market ? In the *now rationed* case, i.e. where we fix labour at the initial (rationed or unrationed) level, we consider also the effects of a change of the restricted level of labour.

The simulation results are contained in tables 1 and 2. Table 1 is based on unrationed optimal starting values for consumption, fertility and labour, whereas table 2 uses levels which are calculated from the restricted model. The starting values for consumption and fertility are given at the bottom of each table, and are of own interest. This allows us to study the effects of a 1% change of the exogenous variables, i.e. we list the responses in % of the endogenous variables: consumption, fertility and labour.

With respect to the interpretation of the price and income effects in the unrationed model with restricted starting values, it should be noted that these effects reflect the reaction to the change in price and income, *as well as* the consequences of lifting the rationing constraint. But it is also clear that the reactions of an individual differ quite substantially depending on het assumed starting position.

Table 1. Preferences and policy simulations: 1% changes of exogenous
variables with *unrestricted* optimal starting values *.

		$\mu=0.2$	$\mu=0.3$	$\mu=0.5$	$\mu=0.7$	$\mu=0.8$
		Exogenous change: +1% price of kid's resources				
Unrationed	C	-0.597	-0.500	-0.233	-0.048	-0.015
model	K	-0.015	-0.048	-0.233	-0.500	-0.597
	L	0.121	0.140	0.167	0.104	0.063
Rationed	C	-0.683	-0.643	-0.512	-0.317	-0.211
model	K	0.006	0.013	0.047	0.128	0.188
		Exogenous change: +1% price effect of wage				
Unrationed	C	0.560	0.455	0.163	-0.038	-0.074
model	K	-0.983	-0.947	-0.746	-0.455	-0.349
	L	5.693	2.250	0.481	0.094	0.043
Rationed	C	0.596	0.753	0.893	1.000	1.061
model	K	-0.006	-0.015	-0.081	-0.404	-0.943
		Exogenous change: +1% non-labour income				
Unrationed	C	0.403	0.500	0.767	0.952	0.985
model	K	0.985	0.952	0.767	0.500	0.403
	L	-5.753	-2.307	-0.551	-0.178	-0.132
Rationed	C	0.410	0.260	0.153	0.128	0.127
model	K	-0.004	-0.005	-0.014	-0.052	-0.113
		Exogenous change: +1% rationed labour				
Rationed	C	0.714	1.022	1.671	2.581	3.103
model	K	-0.178	-0.438	-1.671	-6.023	-12.411
		Calculated optimal starting values for consumption and kids				
Both	C	0.079	0.142	0.348	0.632	0.770
models	K	4.233	3.479	1.916	0.783	0.433
	L	0.145	0.290	0.582	0.780	0.836

* Starting values of exogenous variables and parameters are:
  $\gamma=0.5$, $\beta=0.2$, $\alpha=0.1$, M=0.1, W=1.0, P=1.0.

Table 2. Preferences and policy simulations: 1% changes of exogenous
variables with *restricted* optimal starting values *

		$\mu=0.2$	$\mu=0.3$	$\mu=0.5$	$\mu=0.7$	$\mu=0.8$
		Exogenous change: +1% price of kid's resources				
Unrationed	C	-1.199	-0.660	-0.228	-0.043	0.015
model	K	0.015	-0.043	-0.228	-0.660	-1.199
	L	0.052	0.077	0.228	0.626	1.132
Rationed	C	-0.559	-0.559	-0.559	-0.559	-0.559
model	K	0.033	0.033	0.033	0.033	0.033
		Exogenous change: +1% price effect of wage				
Unrationed	C	0.558	0.372	0.223	0.159	0.140
model	K	-0.578	-0.661	-0.925	-1.542	-2.313
	L	0.516	0.604	0.862	1.448	2.178
Rationed	C	0.860	0.860	0.860	0.860	0.860
model	K	-0.050	-0.050	-0.050	-0.050	-0.050
		Exogenous change: +1% non-labour income				
Unrationed	C	-0.199	0.340	0.772	0.957	1.015
model	K	1.015	0.957	0.772	0.340	-0.199
	L	-0.948	-0.923	-0.772	-0.374	0.132
Rationed	C	0.172	0.172	0.172	0.172	0.172
model	K	-0.010	-0.010	-0.010	-0.010	-0.010
		Exogenous change: +1% rationed labour				
Rationed	C	1.452	1.452	1.452	1.452	1.452
model	K	-1.143	-1.143	-1.143	-1.143	-1.143
		Calculated optimal starting values for consumption and kids				
Both	C	0.275	0.275	0.275	0.275	0.275
models	K	2.362	2.362	2.362	2.362	2.362

* Starting values of exogenous variables and parameters are:
$\gamma=0.5$, $\beta=0.2$, $\alpha=0.1$, M=0.1, W=1.0, P=1.0, L=0.5.

A central issue is the relevance of preferences, which is measured by μ in our model. μ varies in the range $(0,1)$, and $\mu=0.5$ gives equal weight to both activities, consumption and fertility. In tables 1 and 2, we present experiments with $\mu=(0.2, 0.3, 0.5, 0.7, 0.8)$. In all cases, we chose wealth M=0.1, real wage rate W=1.0, relative price of goods devoted to children P=1.0, $\alpha=0.1$, $\beta=0.2$, and $\gamma=0.5$. The calculated optimal starting values for consumption and kids, which are given at the bottom of each table illustrate our first central finding: in the labour constraint case, *preferences play no role* in determining individual decisions; consumption is at 0.275 and fertility at 2.362. This is also true for the *rationed model* with rationed starting values, regardless of which exogenous variable has been changed (see table 2). However, this is not true for the *rationed model with unrestricted starting values* (see table 1), where preferences determine the starting values, but *absolute changes* (in contrast to percentage changes in table 1) do not depend on starting values and, therefore, not on preferences. Note also that with unrestricted starting values, an increase of μ (more weight given to consumption) yields a positive impact on consumption and a negative effect on fertility for exogenous changes of the price of kid's resources and non labour income, where the price effect of wage has the opposite finding.

A 1% increase in the price of kid's resources exhibits a largely negative effect on consumption, independent of the regime and the kind of starting values. Only in the case of strong preferences for consumption (table 2, $\mu=0.8$), there are positive effects in the unrationed model with restricted starting values. Fertility is positively affected in the rationed models; however, the elasticities are largely negative in the unrationed cases. If the starting values are derived from the restricted model and family preferences are strong (table 2, $\mu=0.2$), the effects can be positive. In table 2, the labour supply responses in the unrationed model are positive, increasing in strength as the preference for consumption increases. However, this is not as clear-cut in table 1 though all effects are positive.

The price effect on fertility of a 1% increase in the wage rate turns out to be negative, though the size (in absolute terms) of the elasticities vary substantially in the rationed model with unrestricted starting values (table 1, price effect of wage, unrationed model, K: -0.006 to -0.943) and in the unrationed model with rationed starting values (table 2, price effect of wage, unrationed model, K: -0.578 to -2.313). The elasticities are stronger the larger consumption preferences are in the rationed model with unrestricted starting values (table 1, price effect of wage, rationed model) and in the unrationed model with restricted starting values (table 2, price effect of wage, unrationed model), but this result is reversed in the unrationed model with unrestricted starting values (table 1, price effect of wage, unrationed model). The consumption responses are for the most part positive. These results naturally depend on the choice $\beta > \alpha$, which implies that kids are more time-intensive than consumption. The labour supply response to the wage increase is positive, as in the standard model. However, the size of the responses greatly depends on preferences and starting values. With unrestricted starting values, this magnitude of the labour supply response to wage is declining with rising consumption preferences, whereas this finding is reversed for rationed starting values (table 2, unrationed model, K).

A key issue is the effect of potential income on fertility, consumption and labour supply. Equation (9) states a condition under which fertility is negatively affected by an increase of income; this is the situation where the *positive initial* income effect is over-compensated by an *endogenous price-effect* caused by the increased income. It was difficult to find such a situation in various simulations which had to be consistent with utility maximization. Table 1 shows that fertility is positively affected by income in the unrationed model with unrestricted starting values, and the effect declines in size with rising consumption preferences. However, fertility is negatively affected by income as soon as we are in the rationed regime, independent of the nature of the starting values (see tables 1 and 2). It is worth noting that fertility responses to income are more negative with larger consumption preferences in the rationed model with unrestricted starting values (see table 1). Furthermore, the unrationed model with restricted starting values (see table 2) gives ambiguous results: fertility responses are positive with lower consumption preferences, but negative with very high consumption preferences (μ=0.8). The latter finding follows from equation (9).

Consumption responses to income are mostly positive, with an exception of high family preferences (μ=0.2) in the unrationed model with restricted starting values. Labour supply reacts largely negatively to an increase in income: only high consumption preferences drive the elasticity to be positive in the case of restricted starting values, which follows indirectly from the negative fertility response to income due to equation (9) (see table 2). Note further that labour is less elastic the larger consumption preferences are in the case with unrestricted starting values (see table 1).

Tables 1 and 2 further contain the responses to a 1% increase of rationed labour. In both cases, fertility reacts negatively and consumption reacts positively. For unrationed optimal starting values, the elasticities for both consumption and fertility rise substantially in absolute terms with increasing consumption preferences (see table 1).

As extensive simulations show (see Zimmermann and De New, 1990, for a more complete review of the findings), results are fairly stable with respect to changes in the parameters γ, α and β. A notable exception is the rationed labour case where fertility effects are zero for $\alpha=0.0$ for the rationed model with restricted or unrestricted starting values; only a change of rationed labour affects fertility. This result can be easily understood by studying figure 2.

9.5. Conclusions

We have shown that even a very simplistic economic model is able to mimic a wide range of observed human behaviour. We do this with only four parameters: one for preferences, one for social norms, and two for home-production technology. Labour and fertility are jointly determined in this model. However, if labour market conditions restrict family decisions, this turns out to be essential in determining human behaviour, especially with respect to fertility. For instance, *preferences play no role in determining fertility* if we use rationed starting values.

Naturally, this does not imply that preferences are, in general, irrelevant. On the contrary, we have shown that they play a decisive role under certain conditions. The point we wish to stress is that one should know the conditions.

Furthermore, we show that fertility decline is a more likely event in the process of economic growth which is correlated with increases in income and wages if labour supply is rationed either by underemployment or by over-employment. Given that labour demand has determined employment in recent years, this seems to be an important finding which deserves further attention.

Part IV
Confrontation of Preferences and Restrictions: the Construction of Theoretical Models

ECONOMIC MODELS OF WOMEN'S EMPLOYMENT AND FERTILITY

John F. Ermisch
National Institute of Economic and Social Research
2 Dean Trench Street
LONDON SW1P 3HE
England

10.1. Introduction

Economists take preferences as given, and are concerned with how changes in the constraints that people face, or limits to their choice, alter their behaviour. Indeed, by observing how behaviour changes with elements of these constraints (e.g. prices), they attempt to make inferences about preferences. This viewpoint is maintained in the discussion that follows. In empirical applications, variation in preferences only appears as unobserved random variables. The discussion of models is limited to those which consider both fertility and employment decisions.

Until recently, most economic models of fertility and women's employment have been *static* in nature. That is, they deal with behaviour in a single, timeless period. That period could be a day, a week, a year, or many years, and it is assumed that decisions made in other periods are exogenous. As childbearing takes place over many years, a natural definition of a period would be the main childbearing ages, perhaps including a range of ages after childbearing, and the focus would be on accumulated behaviour over that part of the life cycle. For example, we could analyse completed family size and whether a woman ever worked during her childbearing ages since marriage, or since her first birth, or worked more than some given amount since marriage or first birth. Alternatively, we could study family size and total months of paid employment during some part of the life cycle, such as the first 10 years of marriage or up to age 40.

Modelling the *dynamics* of life cycle behaviour concerning employment and childbearing is more appealing, but it is much more difficult to obtain theoretical predictions of behaviour, and to estimate the interaction between fertility and employment decisions. In order to make the empirical analysis more tractable, movements into and out of paid employment often are analysed conditional on the ages and the number of children, and similarly, the waiting time to another birth of a given order could be modelled conditional on a woman's employment status and experience. The joint modelling of the series of birth events and employment transitions is, however, likely to be necessary, although it has rarely been attempted. In what follows, examples of these various models are discussed, starting with static models of accumulated behaviour.

10.2. Static models

The model developed by Willis (1973) integrated a large amount of previous research on fertility and women's employment (particularly by Becker (1960), Mincer (1963) and Becker and Lewis (1973)) in a framework in which these are jointly determined. It also provided a foundation for most subsequent research. In this model, the planning period is the "lifetime after marriage", or at least that part of it until the children are adults, and fertility control is perfect.

It is assumed that the characteristics of a child that provide satisfaction to its parents can be aggregated into a good called the "quality" of a child, and that the parents choose the same level of child quality for each child born. Parents combine their time and purchased goods and services to produce child quality. Parents may increase the satisfaction derived from each child by increasing the resources devoted to a child, and a given level of child quality may be obtained with alternative combinations of time and goods.

Parents' own consumption is aggregated into a home-produced good, which is produced by combining consumption time of the mother and purchased goods and services. For simplicity, it is assumed that the father's time does not enter into the production of child quality nor this other home production.

The average wage that a mother earns in the period is assumed to depend on the amount of time she spends in paid employment. This reflects skill acquisition on the job, which increases her pay. The couple faces a lifetime budget constraint, which depends on the total amount of time available to the mother after marriage; her wage rate if she takes paid employment; and the sum of the father's lifetime earnings and non-labour income.

Finally, the couple chooses an allocation of the mother's time and of goods, subject to the budget constraint and the relationships between inputs of time and goods and child quality and other home production, in order to obtain the most preferred combination of number of children, child quality and parental consumption. It could be assumed that the level of child quality is exogenous to the parents. This assumption is consistent with the view that child quality is dictated by societal norms, and a stronger prediction of the effect of income on fertility flows from it. The essentials of the model are not, however, changed by this assumption, although Becker (1981) contends that endogenous child quality is an important element in explaining fertility differentials and changes over time.

Completed family size, whether the mother takes paid employment or not after marriage, and her lifetime labour supply and wage if she does, are each endogenous variables in this model. Each depends on the sum of the husband's lifetime income and non-labour income, which shall be called the couple's *"wealth"* for short, and a woman's earning capacity at marriage, which shall be called her *"initial wage."* The wage that the wife would require to take employment is her *"reservation wage."* The larger the wife's initial wage, the more likely that it exceeds the reservation wage, so that she is more likely to take a job after marriage. Because the reservation wage increases with the couple's wealth, the probability of taking a job varies inversely with the couple's wealth. Given that she takes a job, the mother's lifetime labour supply is larger the higher is her initial wage and the lower the couple's wealth. Furthermore, her average wage increases with her labour supply.

While the mother's participation in paid employment and labour supply are, therefore, relatively straightforward in the model, the relationship between fertility and couple's wealth and initial wages is more complicated. Its source, however, is a simple implication of the model: *the demand for children depends on their cost and the couple's wealth.* If, as is plausible, children are more intensive in mother's time (relative to purchased goods and services) than other home production, then the opportunity cost of children increases with a mother's price of time, and higher cost reduces the demand for children. If she takes paid employment, her price of time is her wage; if she does not, it is her reservation wage.

An important implication of this model is that the form of the demand for children by couples in which the mother takes a job after marriage is different from that by couples with only one earner. For the former, a higher initial wage increases the cost of children, and while it also increases the couple's income, it is unlikely that the income effect dominates its impact on cost; thus, a higher initial wage reduces the demand for children. Higher wealth increases the demand for them when child quality is exogenous, but it could have the opposite effect if it is endogenous. Among couples in which the wife is not employed after marriage, the initial wage has no effect on the demand for children, and higher wealth raises the cost of children by increasing the mother's reservation wage. Thus, in these one-earner couples, higher wealth has an algebraically smaller impact than in two earner couples and could reduce fertility, even when child quality is exogenous.

In which of these two groups a couple falls depends on the endogenous employment participation decision. We can express the expected fertility of a couple as a weighted average of the demand for children in each of the two groups with the probability of the mother taking a job and its complement as weights. As this probability depends on the initial wage and the couple's wealth, a non-linear, "interaction" model for fertility emerges. This non-linearity means that the effects of initial wage and couple's wealth on fertility vary in strength and in sign with the levels of these variables.

In particular, at higher levels of couple's wealth, the effect of wealth on fertility is less positive (or more negative), and the impact of the initial wage is less negative, because fewer couples have two earners at higher levels of wealth. At higher levels of the wife's initial wage, the impact of couple's wealth on fertility is more positive (less negative) and the impact of the initial wage is more negative, because it is more likely that a couple has two earners. While the theory is imprecise about whether there is a range of wealth and initial wage in which higher wealth has a negative impact on family size, the impacts of wealth and initial wage at different levels of these which are suggested by the theory are illustrated in table 1.

For example, among couples whose wealth is high and the wife's initial wage is low, few wives would work, so that the wife's potential wage would have no impact on their fertility and higher couple's wealth would be associated with a higher cost of children as well as having a wealth effect. In contrast, most wives who can command a high wage and are in couples with low wealth would take a job, so that a higher wage raises the cost of children while higher couple's wealth does not affect the cost of children and tends to increase fertility.

The application of this model to changes over time was the source of the hypothesis, put forward by Butz and Ward (1979), that fertility switched from being correlated postively with real wages to being correlated negatively as women's participation in paid employment increased. That is, the impact of increases in women's real wages on fertility became more negative as their participation rate increased, and while the effect of men's earnings would become more positive, the former change dominated. This interaction model is also consistent with a J- or U-shaped relationship between a husband's income and fertility if there is positive assortative mating regarding husband's income and wife's initial wage. At higher levels of wealth and wage, more wives take a job, making it possible that the effect of income moves from negative to zero to positive as wealth increases. If, however, the income effect of higher wealth dominates its effect on the cost of children in one-earner couples, higher wealth would increase fertility at all levels of wealth.

Table 1. Suggested impacts of independent variables on family size

Independent variable:	couple's wealth		wife's initial wage	
Level of wife's initial wage	Level of Wealth "Low"	"High"	Level of wealth "Low"	"High"
"Low"	?	-	?	0
"High"	+	?	-	?

While this model may have had explanatory power in the 1950s and 1960s, when married women participated in paid employment less, it appears less relevant today. For instance, in Britain, at least 95 per cent of women born in 1946 worked sometime after marriage. Even if participation in paid employment is defined in a narrower way, such as worked more than X months in the first Y years of marriage, a very large percentage of couples would come into the two-earner group above. Application of Willis' model to this situation suggests that in most couples a higher initial wife's wage would be associated with lower completed fertility and couples with higher wealth would tend to produce a larger family. While evidence is presented below to support these propositions, a different sort of interaction model proposed by Ermisch (1989) now appears more appropriate. This model builds on the foundations of Willis' model. In it, couples choose explicitly a combination of mother's time and *purchased child care* (eg. child-minders, nannies) for the care and rearing of children. Willis' model includes purchased child care in the composite input of purchased goods and services to child quality, thereby concealing some of the implications of this choice. Here it is assumed that while time for child care and rearing can be purchased outside the household, it is not a perfect substitute for the mother's time, and as more child care time is purchased, additional purchased time becomes a poorer substitute for mother's time.

As long as the mother uses some outside child care while rearing her children, a higher price of child care lowers fertility. The effect of the mother's initial wage is more complicated, even though the model assumes that all women take a job sometime after marriage. The model implies that even if children are more time intensive than other home production and that higher income has a relatively small impact on fertility, a higher initial wage could increase fertility if purchased time for child care and rearing is a large enough proportion of child care time. Because it raises this proportion, a lower price of child care makes it more likely that a woman's initial wage has a *positive* effect on family size.

There is a tendency for the impact of a mother's initial wage on family size to vary with the level of her wage, as well as the price of market child care. At low wages (and high prices of child care), it is more likely that no child care is purchased. In these circumstances, all time employed in the care and rearing of children is provided by the mother, making it likely that higher mother's wages reduce family size. At somewhat higher levels of wages, child care is also purchased in the market. In these circumstances, a higher wage tends to reduce the share of mother's time in the cost of a child, creating a tendency for the impact of mother's wages on family size to become less negative (or more positive) at higher levels of wages. Easier substitution between purchased child care and mother's time increases the likelihood that this occurs.

At very high levels of wages, some women would mainly use purchased child care, reducing their input to child care to a minimum. In this situation, a higher wage does not affect the cost of children. Thus, a higher wage only has an income effect, leading to a larger family size. More women are likely to be in this situation as the level of wages increases.

Thus, the main new implication of this variant of Willis' model is that while it is likely that mother's wages have a negative effect on family size at low to moderate levels of wages, their negative impact is predicted to attenuate as her wages rise, or the price of child care falls. The impact of the price of child care on fertility displays a similar interaction with wages, becoming more negative as wages rise, and less negative as the price of child care rises.

But while the price of child care can vary independently of a woman's initial wage in a cross-section, average women's wages and the price of child care move together over time, because labour, particularly women's labour, is the main input in market child care. Thus, increases in women's average wages over time increase the price of child care and the mother's wage, thereby raising the cost of children and reducing fertility. In contrast, in a range in which their wage is high relative to the price of child care, and in some societies (Sweden, for example) this could be a large range, women with a higher wage would have higher fertility.

Estimates of an econometric model of family size of British women at their 15th wedding anniversary, based on this theory, support a diminishing negative impact of a wife's wage at the start of marriage on family size (see table 2: W is the predicted wage at the start of marriage, based on a woman's work experience and education at marriage; R is a measure of husband's "permanent" earnings; and AGEM is age at marriage). Indeed, the impact of the wage is positive for women in the top 5 per cent of the wage distribution (the coefficients of W and W^2 in table 2 imply that the impact of higher wages is positive for women having the potential of earning $2.19 per hour or more at marriage, and such women are in the top 5 per cent of the potential wage distribution; for further details, see Ermisch, 1989).

The theory also implies an equation for women's labour supply after marriage, and such an equation is estimated, in which labour supply is defined as months employed during the first 15 years of marriage (see table 2). A clear implication of this and Willis' model is that the laboursupply equation does not contain *the number of children, because this is endogenous in the model.* When the labour-supply equation in table 2 is re-estimated with the number of children born in the first 15 years of marriage (inappropriately) included as an explanatory variable, it is not surprising to find that it has a large negative coefficient and the R of the equations is increased by a factor of about 8. The elasticities of women's paid employment after marriage with respect to women's potential wage (W) and husband's earnings (R) are 30-40 per cent smaller in size in this specification (see Ermisch, 1989). The smaller elasticities suggest, informally, that the effects of women's wage and husband's earnings on paid employment in table 2 operate in part, but not fully, through their effect on fertility and its corresponding demands on women's time.

In these static models, in which fertility is demand-determined with perfect certainty, there is clearly no reason to include family size in labour supply equations. It would be analogous to including the number of refriger- ators as an "explanatory" variable in an equation for the demand for food. Both variables reflect (unobserved) preferences, and the inclusion of family size produces biased estimates of wage and income effects. One apparent "solution" would be to use an instrumental variable (i.e. an exogenous variable highly correlated with fertility) for fertility rather than its actual value, but what exogenous variables can be used to identify its coefficient ? The only ones suggested by the model should be in the labour supply equation, and to omit one in order to identify the fertility coefficient is arbitrary. Furthermore, as Rosenzweig and Wolpin (1980) point out, no additional information is provided that we could not have obtained by including the identifying variable itself in the labour supply equation (i.e. estimating the conventional labour supply equation, like that in table 2).

Analyses of women's labour "lifetime" supply that interpret the coeffi- cients of the number and ages of children as structural parameters assume (at least implicitly) that these do not enter household preferences or that births are purely random and exogenous. The latter would be the case if couples have no control over their fertility, making births wholly "supply-determined." While fertility is subject to control through contraception, it is undoubtedly imperfect. Unplanned births occur, and these may affect subsequent behaviour, including women's labour supply. These considerations lead us to dynamic models, which are the subject of the next section.

Table 2. Estimates of family size equation and wife's labour supply equation.

Equation:	Family size equation		Wife's labour supply	
Dependent variable:	family size at 15 years of marriage *		months paid employment in first 15 years of marriage **	
Constant	3.845	(7.44)	14.55	(0.60)
W ($)	-1.295	(2.11)	99.62	(3.46)
W^2	0.296	(1.78)	-20.17	(2.85)
R ($1000)	0.091	(3.23)	-3.86	(2.70)
Education:				
A-level or above	0.373	(2.42)	-15.65	(2.21)
O-level	0.093	(0.93)	-16.27	(3.21)
Other	-0.020	(0.23)	-4.05	(0.95)
Marriage Year:				
Before 1945	0.027	(0.22)	-18.65	(3.02)
1945-1949	-0.237	(2.98)	-19.47	(4.77)
1950-1954	-0.014	(0.18)	-12.16	(3.15)
1955-1959	0.008	(0.10)	-6.01	(1.62)
AGEM (years)	-0.070	(5.83)	-0.62	(0.95)
	μ_1	0.898	R^2	0.030
	μ_2	2.009	SE	53.76
	μ_3	2.820	F	4.45
	logL	-2245.4	N	1595

*   Ordered probit estimates; absolute value of asymptotic t-ratio in paren-
     theses. The μ's are threshold parameters in the ordered probit model.
**   Ordinary least squares estimates; absolute value of t-ratio in paren-
     theses. Mean of dependent variable is 67.75.

10.3. Dynamic models

It is on the basis of these unexpected outcomes that we may want to include some measure of fertility in labour supply equations. For instance, if fertility control is costly, then the model should include its cost (which, in effect, reduces the price of childbearing), or the determinants of it, in the labour supply and fertility equations. If it is omitted from these equations, estimates of the other parameters will be biased. But if we lack a measure of it, then some measure of *exogenous* variation in fertility yields information about the response of labour supply to the cost of fertility control relative to the response of fertility to contraceptive costs, as Rosenzweig and Wolpin (1980) demonstrate.

They use twin first births as such a measure, and show that mothers with "twins first" participate in paid employment less than other mothers early in the life cycle, but this appears to be compensated by higher participation later, with apparently little effect on lifetime labour supply. Also, while the life cycle pattern of fertility is altered by an unexpected birth, completed family size hardly changes. Such a compensatory life cycle labour supply response to an unexpected birth is confirmed by a model of the "supply of births" developed by Rosenzweig and Schultz (1985). In their dynamic model, couples choose, in each period, whether to use (imperfect) fertility control or not, the wife's labour supply, and parental consumption in order to obtain the best sequence of births, family size, parental consumption and wife's home time over the remaining periods, subject to the existing family size, the budget constraint in each period (there is no borrowing nor lending), and reproduction "technology." The budget depends on the wife's wage rate, the husband's income, the cost of fertility control and the per-period cost of a child. The reproduction technology expresses the probability of a birth as a sum of a couple-specific fixed component of fertility supply (e.g. fecundity), an unanticipated (serially uncorrelated) component and the impact of fertility control when used. Couples can only change the probability of a birth by altering fertility control.

As is common with these dynamic models with a sequence of decisions, the theoretical model does not produce strong predictions. It does, however, suggest that if children and mother's home time are strong complements (equivalent to the production of child quality being relatively time intensive in Willis' model), unanticipated excess fertility would tend to reduce labour supply and persistent excess fertility, say because of higher fecundity, would have a stronger negative effect on labour supply. The model also suggests that using the actual number of children born at a particular life cycle stage instead of "fertility supply" overestimates the labour supply response to exogenous fertility changes, particularly in the case of response to unantici- pated births, becauses differences between couples in preferences are confounded with supply-side differences in fertility.

From monthly data on couples' conceptions and use of different contra- ceptives, Rosenzweig and Schultz estimate how these components of fertility supply and the exogenous variables suggested by the budget constraint affect contraceptive choice, actual fertility and wife's earnings and labour supply, of which we focus on the last. The empirical estimates confirm the predictions concerning the effect of exogenous differences in fertility supply. A persis- tently higher chance of conception appears to reduce labour supply by an increasing amount over the life cycle, while an unanticipated birth initially reduces it, but within a few years increases it by a roughly similar amount.

This analysis demonstrates the importance of exogenous variation in fertility, associated with imperfect and costly contraception, for women's labour supply. But most data would not allow the construction of exogenous fertility supply. An alternative is to model jointly the sequence of births and women's labour supply, taking into account unobserved, persistent differ- ences between couples in preferences and imperfect fertility control. That is the approach taken by Hotz and Miller (1988).

In their theoretical model, children of a particular age require fixed inputs of maternal time and purchased goods and services. Thus, the "quality" of children is exogenous, and there is no substitution between maternal time and goods and services, nor economies of scale in the rearing of children. Parental consumption is produced by a combination of mother's home time other than child care and purchased goods and services, but it also depends on a couple-specific fixed component. The mother's wages are assumed to be indepen- dent of her experience in employment, although allowance is made for a woman- specific "permanent wage." There is no access to capital markets, neither for borrowing nor lending. Thus, parents face a sequence of period by period budget constraints, with husband's income plus wife's earnings equal to expenditures in each period.

It is assumed that parental pleasure from their offspring varies with the child's age. The parents choose whether to contracept or not and the mother's allocation of time in order to obtain the best expected sequence of births and parental consumption, subject to the birth history so far and the constraints just mentioned. Clearly parents can only influence the probability of a birth in any period through their contraceptive decisions.

The model's predictions concerning the effect of a woman's wage and her husband's income on her labour supply are the same as in Willis' static model, and are confirmed by estimation of the model (using American data) to be positive and negative, respectively. The estimates indicate that the larger the mother's time commitments to child care, the lower her labour supply, while additional required expenditures on children increase her labour supply. Indeed, the parameter estimates support a decline in maternal time inputs with the age of the child and constancy of expenditures on a child with its age. Thus, an unexpected birth produces an initial large reduction in labour supply, but this effect attenuates as the child ages: labour force participation and working hours increase as the child ages.

Higher husband's income is predicted to increase the probability of a birth in a period. This prediction arises because of the lack of capital markets and exogenous child quality, and the empirical analysis confirms a small positive effect. The model also suggests that, given the mother's age, her husband's income and no difference in parental pleasure with a child's age, the probability of a birth increases with the time since the last birth, and parameter estimates support the hypothesis. The duration pattern emerges because younger children make larger demands on the mother's time, thereby raising the cost of an additional child and reducing the demand for one. The estimates indicate, however, that beyond 3 years the probability of a birth declines with duration since the last birth because of a decline in fertility with age and preferences apparently favouring younger children. Finally, the probability of a birth is predicted to fall with parity because of declining marginal benefits from children, and the empirical analysis confirms this. Thus, an unexpected birth tends to reduce subsequent fertility.

Econometric estimation of a model like this is a formidable task. In this case, empirical analysis is confined to time subsequent to a first birth. It is likely that estimation using the entire birth history would be less consistent with the theoretical model because it predicts that women would wish to start childbearing as soon after marriage as chance would allow (i.e. they would not practice contraception). The actual waiting times to first birth in the USA are too long to be consistent with that prediction. In order to account for these longer waiting times, it is probably necessary to model the interdependency of women's pay and their experience in paid employment and possiblly also the impact of the risk of divorce on the timing of her first birth.

Empirical analysis of the *dynamics* of fertility and women's labour supply are appealing because it concerns real changes in behaviour (e.g. moving into or out of a job). Models of these dynamics highlight the uncertainty caused by imperfect fertility control. They can provide an informal guide to empirical analysis, and under some conditions the empirical model can be relatively easy to estimate. For instance, if it possible to measure all of the salient variables, then, even though the number and ages of children are endogenous, a "hazard regression" model (Cox, 1972) could be estimated for women's labour market transitions *conditional* on the number and ages of children, and similarly a hazard model could be estimated for each of the parity-specific conceptions *conditional* on the labour market status of the woman.

But, of course, the concern about endogenous variables is that they are likely to depend on unobserved influences on choices, particularly preferences, as well as observed ones. In contrast to the classical regression model, even if the omitted influence is uncorrelated with those variables in the model, the coefficients in the hazard models are biased. Furthermore, correlation between an unmeasured trait affecting a woman's employment, say a her "career motivation," and her fertility is an additional source of bias in the measured impacts of children on labour supply. Once such unobserved differences between women are taken into account in the model, its estimation is no longer easy. In this case, childbearing and employment transitions need to be modelled jointly in order to obtain unbiased estimates of the effects of children on employment transitions.

The potential for bias may be seen more clearly if we consider a model of waiting time to another birth. In some recent work with Andrew Hinde, we find that, among married childless women, those not in full-time jobs are much more likely to conceive. These women are a relatively small minority. Again, there is very likely to be an unobservable trait, call it "desire for motherhood," which is negatively correlated with participation in full-time employment, so that the coefficient on employment status is at least partly reflecting this unobserved trait. It is indeed likely that if a randomly chosen woman were given a full-time job, it would probably have little impact on her probability of conception. The minority of married childless women not in a full-time employment are *different*, and their employment status is just one aspect of this.

While incorporating the realistic element of imperfect fertility control and the uncertainty it entails, dynamic models like that of Hotz and Miller simplify the economic part of the model to make it more tractable. For instance, as noted earlier, their model assumes that there is no borrowing or lending, that child quality is exogenous and that a woman's pay is unaffected by her work experience, and, perhaps as a consequence, it is unlikely to account well for the important timing of first birth. These models also produce few predictions. Cigno and Ermisch (1989) have, therefore, taken another approach.

The model of Cigno and Ermisch assumes, like the static models of section 2, perfect birth control and the realization of a lifetime plan made at marriage, but it is dynamic in the sense that it focuses on the optimal timing of births and women's participation in paid employment over marriage. It is assumed that each child requires a minimum amount of maternal time and expenditure immediately after the birth, and a "period" is defined as this minimum amount of mother's time. Above the minimum, goods are perfect substitutes for mother's time, and the quality of a child (as perceived by the parents) can be increased by spending more on him/her. Quality is also allowed to vary with the age of the mother at birth. Women's labour supply profile over marriage is just the mirror image of the birth profile: a woman is in employment in a "period" when she is not having a birth. The wage she can earn is assumed to increase with the amount of time she spends in a job. Parents are assumed able to borrow and lend as they choose at a given interest rate, yielding a lifetime budget constraint. Couples choose the best sequence of births, expenditure on children and parental consumption that satisfies these constraints. The discreteness of births is ignored, but the birth and labour supply profile can be interpreted as a smoothing approximation to the actual distribution of births over the marriage (in reality, imperfect fertility control and uncertainty make a major contribution to smoothing the distribution of births).

The model predicts that births tend to occur predominantly in the earlier part of marriage and that birth intervals increase with order of birth. Effects on birth "tempo" or the speed at which completed family size is reached, must be distinguished from effects on family size. Tempo is predicted to increase, while completed fertility falls, when, *ceteris paribus*, a woman's initial wage (at marriage) or the essential expenditure per child is higher (or subsidies per child are lower), or when she marries later. Higher couple's wealth increases tempo, but has an ambiguous effect on family size because of the quality-quantity interaction. The model also suggests that women with steeper earnings profiles will have a slower tempo of fertility. Econometric analysis of British women's first 10 years of marriage confirms most of these predictions. In particular, women in occupations characterized by steeper earnings profiles tend to have their children later in marriage (and a smaller family according to our estimates), and a higher initial wage is associated with a lower family size and a faster tempo.

In this model, predictions about childbearing patterns entail complementary predictions about labour supply. Thus, for instance, women in jobs with steeper earnings profiles would tend to work more early in marriage, and, all else equal, women with a higher initial wage would work more over their lifetime, but less early in their marriage. In sum, this patently unrealistic model concerning fertility control and the discrete nature of births is more realistic in its treatment of the interaction between women's employment and their wage and of borrowing and lending than the sequential decision-making models. Furthermore, it yields a number of hypotheses that can be tested, and which are generally confirmed. Its drawback is that it does not clearly define a structural model that can be estimated, in contrast to Hotz and Miller (1988).

10.4. Conclusion

Despite the plethora of empirical studies of women's labour supply and fertility, there have been relatively few contributions of new models to guide the empirical analysis since the classic study by Willis (1973). The models discussed are representative of the types of models that have been put forward. For instance, Moffitt's (1984b) model of profiles of life cycle fertility, labour supply and women's wages provides no new predictions, and its features are similar to the models present here; the primary contribution is its econometric estimation. Space limitations preclude a more exhaustive review. All of these models stress the interdependency of women's fertility and labour supply decisions, but those that take into account costly and imperfect fertility control also indicate that unexpected fertility outcomes have an important role to play in labour supply decisions.

In terms of the preference-restrictions-behaviour scheme, these economic models focus entirely on how variation in restrictions, over time or over people, affect women's labour supply and fertility behaviour. In the static models, the restrictions are primarily the couple's lifetime budget constraint. But in dynamic models, earlier fertility and labour supply behaviour restricts future choices. In particular, existing children represent constraints on choices, so that future labour supply and fertility responses to wage opportunities and wealth are conditioned on the number of existing children. Thus, both static and dynamic economic models are easily accomodated by the general scheme stressed in this book, again demonstrating the fruitfulness of using this scheme to organize our thinking about women's labour supply and fertility.

MODELS OF FEMALE LABOUR SUPPLY, WITH SPECIAL REFERENCE TO THE EFFECTS OF CHILDREN[1]

Alice Nakamura and Masao Nakamura
University of Alberta .
Faculty of Business
3-23 Faculty of Business Building
EDMONTON, Alberta T6G 2RG
Canada

11.1. Introduction

Much of the public concern about the growing labour force participation of women centers on feared, or hoped for, effects of the market work of mothers on the well-being of their children. On the one side, there are those who fear that the children of working mothers will not receive the care they need, and that women with jobs will more readily divorce their husbands leading to the breakup of the family units on which children depend. On the other side, it is argued that the earning power of their mothers is the only protection large numbers of children have against poverty when the earnings of their fathers are basically inadequate, when fathers are unemployed or ill for long periods of time, or when fathers financially abandon their children.

Both labour economists and the public also view children as the main reason why women work less than men do. Children must be cared for, and in western society it is the mothers to whom this task has traditionally fallen. Empirical explorations of the impacts of children on female labour supply are hampered by the fact that the labour supply responses of mothers to children are not simple cause-effect reactions to the physical existence of children and their biological needs. Rather theory and observation suggest that these responses are molded by family and economic circumstances, aspirations concerning what parents want for and from their children, and societal beliefs. Also many of the responses of interest are thought to take effect over a time span of years, or even decades. Some of these effects are thought to be

[1] The authors are grateful to the workshop participants, and to Harriet Duleep, Martin Dooley, Greg J. Duncan, Paula England, John Ermisch, John Pencavel, and James Walker for helpful comments on earlier versions of this paper and on a related 1987 working paper titled "Theories and Evidence Concerning the Impacts of Children on Female Labor Supply". This research was supported in part by a grant from the Social Sciences and Humanities Research Council of Canada.

anticipatory in nature. And many involve attitudes and theoretically specified personal attributes, such as "human capital", which are inherently hard to observe.

Child status variables are almost always included in economics studies of female labour supply. In some cases, these variables are included because the research objective is to investigate child-related effects on female labour supply. In other cases, primary interest lies in investigating the labour supply effects of other sorts of factors such as wage rates and taxes. In the context of these studies, child status variable are nuisance factors which must be controlled for in order to obtain appropriate estimates of the effects of interest.

In this paper, several different types of models of female labour supply are reviewed. For each model, attention is paid to the mechanisms by which the impacts of children are allowed for. Static models permitting only contemporaneous effects of included variables are considered in the first part of section 2. Reasons for interest in, and key problems in the implementation of, life cycle models are introduced next. Then direct and indirect child status effects on female labour supply are distinguished.

Models of indirect child status effects are the topic of section 3. The first three parts of this section examine indirect child status effects transmitted via human capital investment decisions. The fourth part of section 3 focusses on the key role of hypothesized wage impacts on female labour supply in theories of indirect child status effects. Models providing alternative frameworks for the analysis of direct child status effects are the topic of section 4. These are considered under the headings of models which allow for limited fertility control, models with lifetime budget constraints, and transition models which allow for true state dependence. Conclusions are summarized in section 5.

Empirical tractability is the reason for many of the behavioural simplifications embodied in the models outlined in this paper. However, estimation issues are not dealt with in this paper. The estimation of child status effects on female labour supply is the topic of chapter 12.

11.2. Basic behavioural concepts

Most economic models of female labour supply have the same basic form: a conditional household utility function is maximized subject to time and household budget constraints. Solving this maximization problem yields a *decision rule for determining a woman's labour supply*. For many models of female labour supply, this decision rule can be described in terms of a *reservation wage function*, implied by the maximization problem and defining the minimum wage for which a woman would be willing to work under various circumstances, and an *offered wage* which is what an employer would be willing to pay for an hour (or an additional hour) of this woman's labour. Typically the decision rule has two parts: (1) a woman will work in the current period if her offered wage is greater than or equal to her reservation wage at zero hours of work; and (2) the amount she will work, if she does, is determined so as to equate her reservation wage (which is an increasing function of the amount of time spent in market work) and her offered wage. Thus factors which shift the reservation wage function upward (downward) will tend to decrease (increase) labour supply, while factors which raise (lower) the offered wage will have the opposite effect.

11.2.1. A static, one-period model

The static, one-period model provides a convenient context within which to introduce certain concepts and definitions. By *one-period* what is meant is that a woman's labour supply decisions for the current time period are viewed as the outcome of the maximization of utility for this time period subject to budget and time constraints pertaining to this same period, and without regard to subperiods. Because of the nature of available data, the current time period is often specified to be a year. By *static* what is meant is that current labour supply decisions are not a function of a woman's past (or future) labour supply. Static, one-period models have provided the analytical basis for a large body of applied research on female labour supply. (See, for example, Heckman, 1974b; Nakamura *et al.* 1979; Nakamura and Nakamura', 1981a; and the long list of studies given in Killingsworth, 1983, table 4.3, pp. 193-199.)

In formal terms, for the given time period the woman is assumed to maximize a conditional utility function of the form

$$U = U(X, \ T-H; \ Y, \ Z^*) \tag{1}$$

where X is household consumption of a composite good, T is the total number of hours in the given time period, H is the woman's hours of work, Y is household income excluding the earnings of the wife (sometimes referred to as "other income"), and Z^* is a vector of the current values for predetermined variables arising from previous choices and circumstances. Child status variables are usually included in Z^*. The utility function is maximized subject to the household budget constraint

$$pX = Y + wH \tag{2}$$

and the woman's time constraint

$$0 \le H < T, \tag{3}$$

where p is the unit price of the composite good and w is the wife's *offered wage* rate.

The Lagrangean for this decision problem is

$$G = U(X, \ T-H; \ Z^*) + \lambda_Y(Y + wH - pX) + \lambda_T H, \tag{4}$$

where λ_Y and λ_T are, respectively, an unconstrained and a nonnegative Lagrange multiplier. These Lagrange multipliers can be interpreted as the utility gains associated with relaxing the budget and time constraints, (2) and (3), by one unit each. Hence λ_Y will sometimes be referred to as the marginal utility of other income. The first-order optimality conditions are:

$$U_X - \lambda_Y p = 0, \tag{5}$$

$$- U_L + \lambda_Y w + \lambda_T = 0, \tag{6}$$

$$Y + wH - pX = 0, \tag{7}$$

$$\lambda_T H = 0, \tag{8}$$

where U_X and U_L are the partial derivatives of the utility function with respect to X and L, and where $L = T-H$ is the number of hours of nonmarket work (often referred to in the labour economics literature as "leisure").

From (6) it follows that

$$w = (U_L/\lambda_Y) - (\lambda_T/\lambda_Y) = w^*(H) - (\lambda_T/\lambda_Y), \tag{9}$$

where $w^*(H) = (U_L/\lambda_Y)$ is the *reservation wage*, or the shadow price of a woman's time, at H hours of work.

It follows from the optimality conditions that *a woman will work when her market wage exceeds her reservation wage evaluated at zero hours of work*; that is, when

$$w > w^*(0), \tag{10}$$

or equivalently when

$$\ln w > \ln w^*(0). \tag{11}$$

Moreover the model implies that *a woman who works will choose her hours of work so that her reservation wage evaluated at her actual hours of work equals her offered wage*; that is, a woman will choose her hours of work so

$$w = w^*(H) \text{ when } H > 0. \tag{12}$$

From the definition of the reservation wage it can be seen that w^* depends on H, wH, p, Y and Z^* when H is positive; and on p, Y and Z^* when H is zero.

In empirical applications, it is common to use linear approximations for $\ln w^*(H)$ such as:

$$\ln w^*(H) = \begin{cases} \beta_0 + Z^*\beta_1 + \beta_2 Y + \beta_3 \ln w + \beta_4 H + u^* & \text{if } H > 0 \\ \beta_0 + Z^*\beta_1 + \beta_2 Y + u^* & \text{if } H = 0, \end{cases} \tag{13}$$

where u* is a disturbance term and the β's are parameters to be estimated. It is also common in empirical applications to assume that a woman's offered wage can be expressed as a function of a vector Z of personal characteristics (such as years of schooling) and of variables characterizing labour market conditions (such as the unemployment rate). A typical specification is

$$\ln w = \alpha_0 + Z\alpha_1 + u, \tag{14}$$

where u is a disturbance term and the α's are parameters to be estimated.

Offered wage rates are not usually observed for women who did not work in the given time period. Hence relationships containing the offered wage, such as equation (14), are usually estimated using data for women who worked. For this same reason, a model of the *decision to work* is usually respecified so that the equation to be estimated does not explicitly involve the offered wage. This can be accomplished in the present case by substituting into condition (11) the right-hand side of the expression for $\ln w$ given in (14) and the right-hand side of the expression for $\ln w^*(0)$ given in (13). As a result of these substitutions, a woman's probability of work can be represented as

$$P(H > 0) = P[\ln w > \ln w^*(0)] = F(\phi) \tag{15}$$

where F denotes the cumulative density function for $(u^* - u)$ and

$$\phi = (1/\sigma)[(\alpha_0 - \beta_0) + Z\alpha_1 - Z^*\beta_1 - \beta_2 Y], \tag{16}$$

with σ denoting the standard deviation of $(u^* - u)$.

An equation for a woman's *hours of work* is obtained by equating with $\ln w$ the right-hand side of the expression given in (13) for $\ln w^*(H)$ when H is positive, in accordance with condition (12); and then solving for H. The resulting equation is:

$$H = (1/\beta_4)[(1-\beta_3)\ln w - \beta_0 - Z^*\beta_1 - \beta_2 Y - u^*]. \tag{17}$$

11.2.2. Life cycle models

In real life, women often plan for both careers and children, with these plans stretching over many years. The one-period model cannot incorporate or allow for planning over multiple time periods within a longer time horizon. Mincer was one of the first to draw attention to this shortcoming. Mincer states:

"... the *timing* of market activities during the working life may differ from one individual to another. The life cycle induces changes in demands for and marginal costs of home work and leisure ... There are life cycle variations in family incomes and assets which may affect the timing of labor force participation ..." (Mincer, 1962, p. 68).

In his survey of the literature on the labour supply behaviour of men, Pencavel provides a cogent summing up of the key problems faced in implementing life cycle labour supply models:

"The empirical implementation of the life-cycle model would appear to require a great volume of data: to understand an individual's labor supply today, the economist needs information on prices and wages throughout the individual's life ! In fact, the empirical work on life-cycle labor supply has proceeded by placing sufficient restrictions on the form of the lifetime utility function that the parameters governing the dynamic allocation of consumption and hours can be estimated with relatively little data. To date, there exist two general approaches to this dynamic allocation problem. One derives from the literature on habit persistence and stock adjustment and specifies the individual's utility function in period t as conditional on the individual's consumption and hours of work in the previous period. The notion that the standards by which individuals gauge their welfare are molded by their prior experiences is, of course, an old one. ... Whereas in this specification the lifetime utility function is intertemporally not (strongly) separable, the opposite hypothesis is maintained in the second approach to the individual's life-cycle labor supply problem." (Pencavel, 1986, p. 46).

Thus Pencavel differentiates two classes of life cycle models depending, in formal terms, on whether the utility function is intertemporally (strongly) separable. Gorman captures in words the empirical importance and, indeed, necessity of explicit and implicit *separability assumptions*, and the key role economic theory plays in both motivating and justifying these assumptions. Gorman writes:

"Separability is about the structure we are to impose on our model: what to investigate in detail, what can be sketched in with broad strokes without violence to the facts. Perfect competition and the absence of external economies, which allow us to examine the behaviour of individual firms in isolation; constant returns, permitting us to discuss the structure of a firm's production plans without knowing its size; Samuelson's independence axiom which says that how we use our resources when it shines is independent of how we would have had it rained; and Bergson's Social Welfare Function, based on the sovereignty of self-regarding households; all embodying separability assumptions, whose function is to allow us to examine one aspect of a problem in at least relative isolation from the others, given that we have posed it in terms of appropriate independent variables." (Gorman, 1987, p. 305)

In real life, people's plans for education and training, work, family formation, and expenditure and savings extend over long time periods, though these plans may be revised; and these different sorts of plans are surely interrelated. Yet all tractable life cycle models of female labour supply behaviour explicitly allow for only certain interactions with other types of behaviour, and for only certain types of influences across time periods.

11.2.3. Modelling the impacts of children on female labour supply

Alternative models of female work behaviour can be grouped according to the sorts of child status effects that can be explicitly represented. Hypothesized child status effects can be grouped into two main categories: direct and indirect. The *direct effects* of the time, effort and other resources devoted to having and caring for children are usually modelled as affecting the labour supply of a woman via her reservation wage, which by definition reflects the competing household needs for her time versus the income she could earn.

It is also hypothesized that children affect the amounts and types of human capital that women accumulate, and furthermore that human capital accumulation affects women's offered wage rates which in turn affect their labour supply. These theorized *indirect effects* of children on female labour supply are the subject of the following section. Section 4 is devoted to theories and models allowing for direct, reservation wage-related effects of children.

11.3. Indirect effects of children on female labour supply

All of the theories concerning indirect, human capital-related effects of children on female labour supply begin with the presumption that most women plan to and do have children. Moreover it is assumed that most women plan to and do supply less market labour during their active child bearing and rearing years. The theories differ in terms of whether effects on the amount or the type of human capital investment are emphasized, and depending on who is viewed as choosing whether or not to make (and pay for) these investments.

11.3.1. Human capital investment decisions of women and their families

If wives devote less time to market work than their husbands while bearing and rearing children, they will accumulate less job experience than their husbands. Job experience is usually thought to contribute to an individual's stock of job-related human capital.

Also training in job-related skills is usually obtained in the hope of enhancing one's job-related human capital. Mincer and Polachek (1974, p. 401) argue that "since job-related investment in human capital commands a return which is received at work, the shorter the ... actual [or expected] duration of work experience, the weaker the incentives [of individuals] to augment job skills over the life cycle." Following this line of argument, the investment decisions of couples with children should tend to increase the wage rates of the husbands relative to the wives. In turn, the generally higher offered wage rates of the husbands should lead them to specialize more in market work and wives to specialize more in household work even when the child bearing and rearing years are over. An implication of these theories is that the cumulative investment effects of the child-related roles of women should cause the offered wage gap between wives and husbands to widen over the course of the life cycle.

Arguments concerning linkages among children, labour supply and human capital investment have been expanded to encompass anticipatory behaviour prior to marriage and even parental choices concerning the education and training of children. According to Mincer and Polachek:

> "Prospective discontinuity may well influence many young women during their prematernal employment ... to acquire less job training than men with comparable education ..." (Mincer and Polachek, 1974, p. 404).

And Becker argues:

> "Since specialized investments begin while boys and girls are very young ..., they are made prior to full knowledge of the biological orientation of children, which is often not revealed until the teens or even later. If only a small fraction of girls are biologically oriented to market rather than household activities, and if only a small fraction of boys are biologically oriented to household

activities, then in the face of no initial information to the contrary, the optimal strategy would be to invest mainly household capital in all girls and mainly market capital in all boys until any deviation from this norm is established." (Becker, 1981, p. 24).

That is, Becker argues that rational parents, and others in society as well, will invest less in the job-related education of girls than of boys. If behaviour of this sort is widespread, then, even before marriage and children, young women will tend to be at a disadvantage versus young men in terms of their accumulated stock of job-related human capital.

11.3.2. Atrophy and wage appreciation theories of occupational choice

Another sort of anticipatory theory focusing more on the type of job-related human capital investment is developed in Polachek's papers (1976, 1979, 1981). He specifies a model of occupational choice in which it is assumed that by choosing the kinds as well as the amounts of human capital investments, individuals choose occupations with characteristics that will maximize their expected lifetime earnings. In the formal derivation of his model, Polachek (1981, p. 16) represents lifetime earnings as the product of years of work, the rental rate per unit of human capital of a given type, and the amount of human capital of the given type. It is assumed that an individual's stock of human capital "atrophies" during years of home time at a rate determined uniquely by the kind of human capital that the individual has accumulated. Thus for any given number of years of home time, the loss of human capital will be greater in those occupations characterized by higher atrophy rates.

Polachek concludes that women will tend to choose different occupations than men because most women anticipate that their labour force participation will be more intermittent. In particular, most women are expected to prefer occupations with lower atrophy rates. Moreover, among women, those who anticipate more intermittency in their labour force participation are expected to be more interested in choosing occupations with lower atrophy rates.

A related theory of female occupational choice is suggested by H. Zellner (1975). She notes that jobs with steep earnings-experience profiles are thought to have low starting wages because employees pay some portion of the specific training costs associated with these jobs through foregone earnings. She argues that women who anticipate dropping out of the work force to raise children will not select jobs of this sort because, when these jobs are held for only short periods, the realized appreciation in earnings will not provide adequate compensation for the lower starting wages. According to Zellner's theory, therefore, women will tend to be found in occupations characterized by relatively high starting wage rates, but low rates of wage appreciation with increased work experience.

11.3.3. Human capital investment practices of employers

If women work intermittently, they will accumulate fewer hours of job experience than most men. Both human capital and more institutionally based screening and seniority arguments suggest that rational employers will pay relatively lower wage rates to workers with less actual experience, and also that employers will be less inclined to make training investments in workers who are expected to supply relatively less labour in future time periods. Becker explains:

> "If a firm had paid for the specific training of a worker who quit ..., its capital expenditure would be partly wasted, for no further return could be collected. ... The willingness of ... firms to pay for specific training should, therefore, closely depend on the likelihood of labor turnover." (Becker, 1975, p. 29).

The theory of statistical discrimination suggests that even women who do not, and may never, have children may still be passed over by employers with no personal biases against working women when it comes to opportunities for employer-subsidized training. (See Aigner and Cain, 1977; and the classic paper of Phelps, 1972). Bielby and Baron provide a verbal description of the concept (in their words, the model) of statistical discrimination with respect to the employment of women:

> "The model assumes employers perceive that on average the marginal productivity of men and women differ for a given line of work. For example, within a specific occupation, women may be more likely to quit their jobs. If an employer incurs significant turnover costs due to the expense of finding and training new employees, the expected net contribution of the average female job applicant is less than that of an otherwise comparable male applicant. The model also assumes that it is unduly costly to ascertain these differences among individual male and female job applicants. For example, employers may be unable to devise any procedure for screening individual applicants with respect to quit propensity or work commitment. ... Group differences may in fact be small relative to variation within groups; there may be many female applicants with lower quit propensities and

greater work commitment than the average male applicant. But if
employers are unable to obtain this information for individual
applicants, expected profits are maximized by segregating workers by
sex. Females will be allocated to jobs with low turnover costs. ...
Moreover, statistical discrimination produces inequities between men
and women in wages and other career outcomes." (Bielby and Baron,
1986, pp. 761-766).

11.3.4. Wage effects on labour supply

The indirect effects of children have been defined as child-related effects
on labour supply transmitted via the offered wage. So far we have reviewed a
number of child-related, human capital investment factors that are presumed
to lower the wage rates of women. If this is the case, then the indirect
effects of children on female labour supply will be negative if there is a
positive relationship between women's offered wage rates and their labour
supply, and will be positive otherwise.

As explained in section 2, economic models of female labour supply
typically imply that a woman will work in a given time period if her offered
wage exceeds her reservation wage evaluated at zero hours of work. Clearly
then, these models also imply that factors which decrease (increase) a woman's
offered wage will decrease (increase) the probability that she will engage in
market work in the given time period.

The implied nature of the effect of a wage change on the hours of work
of a working woman is more complex. Mincer explains:

"On the assumption that leisure time is a normal good, the standard
analysis of work-leisure choices implies a positive substitution
effect and a negative income effect on the response of hours of work
supplied to variations in the wage rate. An increase in the real wage
rate makes leisure time more expensive and tends to elicit an
increase in hours of work. However, for a given amount of hours
worked, an increase in the wage rate constitutes an increase in
income, which leads to an increase in purchases of various goods,
including leisure time. Thus, on account of the income effect, hours
of work tend to decrease. In which direction hours of work change on
balance, given a change in the wage rate, ... depends on the relative
strengths of the income and substitution effects in the relevant
range." (Mincer, 1962, p. 65).

Two lines of argument have been presented suggesting that, for married women,
the negative income effects on labour supply associated with a wage change may

be weak in comparison with the positive substitution effects. The first of these lines of argument is due to Mincer (1962).

According to Mincer, married women divide their time among work at home, work in the market, and leisure. He assumes that income has a positive effect on the demand for leisure, and hence a negative effect on the total amount of (home and market) work. But in some cases, income earned through market work can be used to purchase substitutes (such as child care and restaurant meals) for work in the home. Mincer concludes that "the lesser the substitutability the weaker the negative income effect on hours of work at home, and the stronger the income effect on hours of work in the market" (p. 65). Nevertheless so long as some substitution is possible between the wife's time and market-produced goods or what Mincer terms "other (mechanical, or human) factors of production at home", it is argued that the income effect associated with a given wage change should be weaker for a married woman than for an otherwise similar married man who is presumed to divide his time only between work in the market and leisure. That is, the income effect associated with a given wage change is assumed to be stronger for husbands because they must give up leisure in order to work longer hours, while wives can increase their market work without necessarily sacrificing their leisure.

The second line of argument concerning the strength of the income effect for working wives is much simpler. Holding hours of work constant, the dollar value of the change in earned income associated with any given wage change will be smaller (larger) the shorter (longer) the hours of work are. Following this line of reasoning, when wives work less than full-time or full-year because of child care and household responsibilities, the income effects associated with any given wage change should be weaker for them than for their husbands who predominantly work longer hours.

If the negative income effects associated with a wage change are weaker for married women who work than for married men (and presumably for unmarried women and unmarried men as well) and if the positive substitution effects are similar for married women and married men, then the relationship between changes in hours of work and wage rates should be more positive for married women than for married men (or for unmarried women or unmarried men). Some have argued on these grounds that the net effect of a wage change on the hours of work of working wives will almost surely be positive, and may possibly be large in magnitude.

11.4. Direct effects of children on female labour supply

As already noted, in order for models of female labour supply to be analyti-
cally and empirically tractable it is necessary to limit the types of effects
that are explicitly allowed for. Hence models of female labour supply allowing
for indirect, human capital-related effects of children usually ignore factors
directly affecting labour supply decisions through women's utility functions
or the household budget constraint. On the other hand, the types of models that
offer the most promise as frameworks for investigating the direct effects of
children on female labour supply usually ignore human capital accumulation
behaviour.

11.4.1. Models which allow for limited fertility control

Hotz and Miller (1988, p. 92) note that most empirical studies of female labour
supply treat children as exogenously imposed constraints. They state that their
analysis "departs from this latter approach by recognizing that such
constraints are chosen by parents indirectly via the contraceptive strategies
they follow over their lifetimes." Parents' contraceptive decisions are characterized by an index function which involves the husband's income, the woman's
time costs for rearing her existing children, monetary expenditures due to
existing children, the woman's birth history (described by dummy variables
indicating the birth years for her children), and an age variable included "to
account for the fact that women at different ages have different market wage
prospects given the age trend in their market wage opportunities" (p. 96). Hotz
and Miller also note that parental desires for children may differ depending
on expectations about the amount of time remaining before the wife reaches
menopause. On a modelling level, therefore, certain aspects of the technology
of child bearing and rearing are explicitly treated in the Hotz-Miller study.
Empirical implementation of this aspect of the model is hampered because the
data utilized by Hotz and Miller contain no information about contraceptive
usage or the monetary costs of caring for existing children, and limited
information about child-related time costs. Nevertheless, a number of
interesting results emerge concerning child-related effects on female labour
supply.

    An earlier study by Rosenzweig and Schultz (1985) more fully develops
the concept that fertility is determined by the dynamic interaction between

the biological capacity to bear children that is stochastic and mostly unaffected by choice behaviour (the supply of births) and the financial resources devoted to birth control (reflecting the demand for births). Placing their study in a historical context, Rosenzweig and Schultz note:

> "Economists have recognized the joint relevance of biological and behavioral factors in determining fertility under a regime of costly fertility control ... , but this perspective has not been suitably incorporated into the empirical study of fertility. In particular, this insight has not been employed in estimating the effectiveness of contraceptive methods, or in estimating the effects of fertility variation on labor supply behavior ..." (Rosenzweig and Schultz, 1985, p. 993).

The Rosenzweig and Schultz study explicitly models contraceptive usage by type. Moreover the data used in this study contain detailed information on the fertility control practices of couples. Differences in the use of fertility control are related to differences among households in fecundity. However, no attention is paid to the time or monetary costs of caring for children, as in the Hotz-Miller study.

As in the Hotz-Miller study, there is no provision for inter-period borrowing or saving. Thus possible effects of a woman's wage offers in other time periods are ignored. Also human capital accumulation decisions are ignored.

11.4.2. Models with lifetime budget constraints

In one-period models, there is no intertemporal borrowing or saving and the household budget constraint must be satisfied in each time period. Hence one-period models cannot provide a framework, for example, for incorporating variations in the timing of children in response to a woman's future expectations about her offered wage rate. Models with lifetime budget constraints could be extended, however, to encompass intertemporal choices of this sort.

Heckman and MaCurdy (1980, 1982) present such a model, which is based on earlier work by Heckman (1974a, 1974b, 1976b) and MaCurdy (1977, 1978). This model is perhaps the most important example so far of the second of the two approaches to implementing life cycle concepts delineated by Pencavel (see subsection 2.2).

A woman is assumed to maximize a lifetime, additively-separable utility function which can be written in a discrete-time form as

$$U = \sum_{t=1}^{N} (1 + s)^{-t} U[X(t), T-H(t)],$$ (18)

subject to the lifetime budget constraint

$$S(0) + \sum_{t=1}^{N} (1 + r)^{-t} [w(t)H(t) - p(t)X(t)] = 0$$ (19)

and the time constraint in each period that

$$0 \leq H(t) < T.$$ (20)

In accordance with the notation used in section 2, for period t, $X(t)$ is household consumption of a composite good with unit price $p(t)$, $H(t)$ is the woman's hours of work, and $w(t)$ is the woman's offered wage rate. T is the total number of hours in a given time period which is presumed the same in all time periods, and (N+1) is the total number of time periods in the person's adult lifetime. Also s, which is the woman's subjective rate of time preference; r, which is the market rate of interest; and $U[\cdot]$, which is a strictly concave single-period utility function, are all assumed to be the same in all time periods. Finally, $S(0)$ is the woman's initial savings and asset holdings (that is, her net worth at the start of period t=0). In this simplest specification of the model, income from other family members (including the husband's earnings) is ignored.

The Lagrangean for this decision problem for periods t = 0, ..., N is:

$$G = \sum_{t=1}^{N} (1 + s)^{-t} \{U[X(t), T - H(t)] + \lambda_T(t)H(t)\} +$$

$$+ \lambda_S(0) \{S(0) + \sum_{t=1}^{N} (1 + r)^{-t} [w(t)H(t) - p(t)X(t)]\},$$ (21)

where $\lambda_S(0)$ is the Lagrange multiplier associated with the lifetime budget constraint (19), and $\lambda_T(t)$ (which must be nonnegative) are the Lagrange multipliers associated with the time constraints (20). Following Killingsworth and Heckman (1986, p. 151), for convenience we define

$$\lambda_S(t) = [(1 + r)/(1 + s)]^{-t} \lambda_S(0).$$ (22)

Then for $t = 0, \ldots, N$, the first-order optimality conditions for this decision problem are:

$$U_x(t) - \lambda_S(t) \, p(t) = 0, \tag{23}$$

$$- U_L(t) + \lambda_S(t) \, w(t) + \lambda_T(t) = 0, \tag{24}$$

$$S(0) + \sum_{t=1}^{L} (1 + r)^{-t} \, [s(t) \, H(t) - p(t) \, X(t)] = 0, \tag{25}$$

$$\lambda_T(t) \, H(t) = 0, \tag{26}$$

where now $L(t) = T-H(t)$ so that $U_L(t)$ is the partial deviative of the utility function for period t with respect to nonmarket time.

From (24) it follows that

$$w(t) = [U_L/\lambda_S(t)] - [\lambda_T(t)/\lambda_S(t)] = w^*[H(t)] - [\lambda_T(t)/\lambda_S(t)], \tag{27}$$

where $w^*[H(t)] = [U_L/\lambda_S(t)]$ is the *reservation wage*, or shadow price of a woman's time, at H hours of work in period t. From (22) and (23), it can be seen that $\lambda_S(t)$ is positive. Hence from the nonnegativity of $\lambda_T(t)$ and condition (26) it follows that

$$w(t) \leq w^*[H(t)] \qquad \text{for } H(t) = 0, \tag{28}$$

$$w(t) = w^*[H(t)] \qquad \text{for } H(t) > 0. \tag{29}$$

Note that in this model $\lambda_S(0)$, which may be interpreted as the marginal utility of the woman's initial net worth, is endogenous just like X(t) and L(t) (and hence also hours of work given by H(t) = T - L(t)). The value of $\lambda_S(0)$ is simultaneously determined along with the values of X(t) and L(t) for t = 1, ..., N, given the values of the exogenous variables (which include S(0) and also w(t) and p(t) for t = 0, ..., N). If the values of $\lambda_S(0)$ are fixed over time for individuals, then the resulting demand functions for X(t) and L(t) are sometimes called "marginal utility of wealth-constant" demand functions; or "Frisch" demand functions following Browning (1982) and Browning *et al.* (1985), and in recognition of Frisch's extensive use of additive utility

functions. An important feature of this class of demand functions is that they
relate decisions in any given period t to variables for other time periods
solely through the Lagrange multiplier associated with the lifetime budget
constraint, denoted here by $\lambda_S(0)$. One implication of this sort of a life cycle
model is that a woman's reservation wage in any given time period depends,
through $\lambda_S(0)$, on her market wage rates in all time periods.

11.4.3. Transition models which allow for true state dependence

The basic assumption underlying the Heckman-MaCurdy model as presented in
their 1980 paper is that the impacts of all past and expected future decisions
and experiences of women that affect their current labour supply decisions can
be captured in a single, unchanging, individual-specific parameter ($\lambda_s(0)$ as
the model is presented in the previous subsection). Heckman and MaCurdy (1980,
p. 56) note that, "Using panel data, one can eliminate the fixed effect, and
hence purge the analysis of unobservable variables that are bound to be correlated with the included variables...."

But suppose that in addition to, or instead of, intertemporal interactions
that can be captured in individual-specific, fixed effects terms, there are
interactions that develop over time in an evolutionary fashion. That is,
suppose there is true state dependence (as contrasted with the spurious state
dependence, sometimes termed *heterogeneity*, that can result from the presence
of individual-specific fixed effects). *True state dependence* means that the
change(s) from one period to the next in the dependent variable(s) of a model
depend in a direct causal sense on the previous value(s) of the dependent
variable(s). (See Heckman, 1981). The final form in which Heckman and MaCurdy
(1980) present their model and the estimation approach they suggest cannot
easily accommodate true state dependence. Yet casual empiricism would suggest
that processes such as learning how to blend work outside the home and
parenting are intrinsically evolutionary in nature, with outcomes that are
revealed through doing and which are often less than perfectly foreseen.

The approach adopted in Nakamura and Nakamura (1985a) can be modified
to allow for true state dependence as well as for individual-specific fixed
effects. The approach is based on reformulating the labour supply model in a
first difference form. First difference formulations of models embodying
inequality decision rules are conceptually more difficult to specify than is
the case for intrinsically linear models.

We begin by adopting the customary specification of the *reservation wage for those who work* as an increasing function of the reservation wage at zero hours of work and of ln w and H (see 13)):

$$\ln w^*(H) = \ln w^*(0) + \beta_3 \ln w + \beta_4 H \text{ if } H > 0. \tag{30}$$

But now the *reservation wage evaluated at zero hours of work* is specified as being given by

$$\ln w^*(0) = \gamma^* \ln w^*(0)_{-1} + \Delta Z^* \beta_1 + \beta_2 \Delta Y + e^*, \tag{31}$$

where a sub minus one indicates that the variable is for the previous time period and a Δ denotes a current-previous period difference. Suppose the parameter γ^* in (31) equals one. In this case, (31) can be obtained directly from the static, one-period specification for $\ln w^*(0)$ given in (13) with e^* redefined as first differences for the original error term. The meaning, in this case, is simply that the reservation wage evaluated at zero hours of work will be the same this period as it was last unless there are random changes, changes in Y, or changes in the values of variables in Z^*. If γ^* is greater than one, then women's reservation wage rates at zero hours of work will tend to rise over time even in the absence of other changes in observable or unobservable factors.

Suppose that the static, one period formulation for the *offered wage* equation given in (14) is also modified as follows to allow for true state dependence:

$$\ln w = \gamma \ln w_{-1} + \Delta Z \alpha_1 + e. \tag{32}$$

The interpretation of (32) is analogous to the interpretation of (31).

Recall that in the static, one-period model the *condition for work* in the current period (given in (11)) is

$$\ln w > \ln w^*(0).$$

Notice that this condition is *not* equivalent to

$$\ln w - \ln w_{-1} > \ln w^*(0) - \ln w^*(0)_{-1}.$$

However, an equivalent *difference version of the condition to work* is given by the following inequality statement:

$$\ln w - \ln w_{-1} > \ln w^*(0) - \ln w_{-1}. \tag{33}$$

From (32) we see that the expression on the left-hand side of (32) can be written as

$$\ln w - \ln w_{-1} = (\gamma-1) \ln w_{-1} + \Delta Z \alpha + e. \tag{34}$$

As for the right-hand side of (33), it can be seen from (31) that

$$\ln w^*(0) - \ln w_{-1} = \gamma^* \ln w^*(0)_{-1} + \Delta Z^* \beta_1 + \beta_2 \Delta Y - \ln w_{-1} + e^*. \tag{35}$$

For those who worked in t-1, we see from (30) that

$$\ln w^*(0)_{-1} = \ln w^*(H)_{-1} - \beta_3 \ln w_{-1} - \beta_4 H_{-1}. \tag{36}$$

Also for those who worked in period t-1 we have the condition that hours of work will be chosen so that

$$\ln w^*(H)_{-1} = \ln w_{-1}. \tag{37}$$

This means that (35) can be rewritten as

$$\ln w^*(0) - \ln w_{-1} =$$

$$= \Delta Z^* \beta_1 + \beta_2 \Delta Y + [\gamma^*(1-\beta_3) - 1] \ln w_{-1} - \gamma^* \beta_4 H_{-1} + e^*. \tag{38}$$

Thus from (34) and (38) it follows that for those who worked in t-1, the *condition for work in period t* given in (33) can be rewritten as

$$[\Delta Z \alpha - \Delta Z^* \beta_1 - \beta_2 \Delta Y + (\gamma - \gamma^*(1-\beta_3)) \ln w_{-1} + \gamma^* \beta_4 H_{-1}] > (e^* - e). \tag{39}$$

This means that for women who worked in the previous period, the *probability of work in the current period* is given by

$$P(H > 0) = F(\phi^D) \tag{40}$$

where F denotes the cumulative standard normal density function if the error terms e^* and e are jointly normally distributed with zero means and constant variances, and where

$$\phi^D = (1/\sigma^D)[\Delta Z\alpha - \Delta Z^*\beta_1 - \beta_2\Delta Y + (\gamma - \gamma^*(1-\beta_3))\ln w_{-1} + \gamma^*\beta_4 H_{-1}] \tag{41}$$

with σ^D denoting the standard deviation of (e^*-e).

The optimal hours of work for those who work and who also worked in t-1 can be found by substituting the right-hand side of (36) into (31), substituting the right-hand side of the resulting expression for $\ln w^*(0)$ into (30), applying the condition for both periods t and t-1 that for those who work the hours of work will be chosen so as to equate the reservation wage with the offered wage (hence $\ln w^*(H) = \ln w$ and $\ln w^*(H)_{-1} = \ln w_{-1}$), and solving for H. The resulting expression for the optimal hours of work is:

$$H = (1/\beta_4)[(1-\beta_3)\ln w - \Delta Z^*\beta_1 - \beta_2\Delta Y - \gamma^*(1-\beta_3)\ln w_{-1} + \gamma^*\beta_4 H_{-1} - e^*]. \tag{42}$$

For those with a work history but who did not work in the previous time period, condition (32) for work might be rewritten as

$$\ln w - \ln w_L > \ln w^*(0) - \ln w_L, \tag{43}$$

where w_L denotes the (real) offered wage for the last job the woman held. This will result in a formulation identical to the one developed in expressions (33) - (41) for women who worked in the previous year, with a sub L substituted throughout for a sub one, and with all differences (denoted by Δ) defined as between current period values and the values in period L, where L is the individual-specific time period when each woman last worked. For women who never worked before, there is no alternative except to estimate the model in levels rather than difference form, ignoring possible fixed effects and true state dependence.

11.5. Conclusions

A sequence of models of female labour supply have been reviewed with attention to mechanisms by which child status effects are, or potentially could be, incorporated. The effects on female labour supply of the time, expenditure and effort needed to bear and raise children are termed *direct child status* effects. The labour supply effects of children due to effects on human capital accumulation transmitted via the wage offers women receive are termed *indirect child status* effects.

There are many reasons for trying to gain a better understanding of the *effects of children on women's offered wage rates*. However, the extent to which it is also important to gain a better understanding of *indirect child status effects on female labour supply, transmitted via women's wage offers*, depends on the extent to which female labour supply is responsive to current period or intertemporal offered wage rates. It is argued in a companion paper (see chapter 12) that the evidence concerning offered wage effects on female labour supply is far from conclusive.

Current period, direct child status effects can be represented in a static, one-period model of female labour supply. Certain types of *intertemporal direct effects* can potentially be allowed for in fixed-effects, life cycle models of female labour supply of the sort presented by Heckman and MaCurdy (1980). Finally, it is argued that an empirically tractable model which can accommodate both *true state dependence and heterogeneity* can be developed along the lines of the first difference model given in Nakamura and Nakamura (1985a). (See also Nakamura and Nakamura, 1985b.) Certain empirical aspects of this sort of a modelling approach are explored more fully in chapter 12.

In much of the earlier literature on female labour supply, it was acknowledged that children do have important effects on female labour supply. However, in most of those studies the child-related effects were treated as nuisance factors which had to be controlled for in order to obtain efficient and consistent estimates of the income and substitution effects of primary interest. Recently there has been more interest in child status effects in their own right. We would hope that this interest will accelerate progress toward developing theoretical models which incorporate increasingly explicit and realistic representations of hypothesized effects of children on the labour supply behaviour of women.

CHILDREN AND FEMALE LABOUR SUPPLY:
A SURVEY OF ECONOMETRIC APPROACHES[1]

Alice Nakamura and Masao Nakamura
University of Alberta
Faculty of Business
3-23 Faculty of Business Building
EDMONTON, Alberta T6G 2R6
Canada

12.1. Introduction

The way in which economists try to learn about economic responses, such as the effects of children on female labour supply, can be broken down into three steps:

1. the consideration of information already available called *a priori* information, including inferences based on what economists believe they know about other aspects of economic behaviour, and the formulation of qualitative, nonparametric behavioural concepts and hypotheses that are usually stated in words;
2. the specification of mathematical models that are consistent with the *a priori* information and which provide parametric representations of the behavioural hypotheses of interest;
3. the use of available data and statistical methods to estimate, and then to test and interpret, the parameters of the specified mathematical models.

Steps 1 and 2 are sometimes viewed as the purview of *mathematical economics*, while step 3 is seen as the domain of *econometrics*. Most textbooks on econometrics deal with the problems of estimating, testing and interpreting the parameters of given, mathematically specified models.

---

[1] The authors are grateful to the workshop participants, and to Harriet Duleep, Martin Dooley, Greg J. Duncan, Paula England, John Ermisch, John Pencavel, and James Walker for helpful comments on earlier versions of this paper and on a related 1987 working paper titled "Theories and Evidence Concerning the Impacts of Children on Female Labor Supply". This research was supported in part by a grant from the Social Sciences and Humanities Research Council of Canada.

The formulation of mathematical models of female labour supply is the topic of a companion paper (chapter 11). The present paper focusses on the estimation of the parameters of models of female labour supply, and, in particular, on the estimation of child-related effects on female labour supply.

The basic behavioural concepts underlying most economic models of female labour supply are summarized in section 2. Also a distinction is drawn between direct and indirect child-related effects on female labour supply. In section 3 the key equations of a static, one-period model of female labour supply are summarized.

One of the insights which emerges from sections 2 and 3 is that the nature of indirect child-related effects on female labour supply depends critically on how the labour supply decisions of women are affected by the wage offers they receive from employers. There is a large body of empirical literature on measuring these wage effects. This literature and related econometric issues are selectively discussed in section 4. Problems concerning the estimation of direct child status effects are the subject of section 5. Conclusions are summarized in section 6.

12.2. Basic behavioural concepts

In most economic models of female labour supply, each woman is viewed as having both an offered wage and a reservation wage. The *offered wage* is defined as what an employer would be willing to pay for an (or another) hour of the woman's time. The *reservation wage* is defined as the amount of money the woman would require to be willing to work one (or one more) hour. Usually it is thought that the more hours a woman works, the more she will value her remaining nonwork hours. Thus the reservation wage is assumed to be an increasing function of hours of market work.

The *decision rules* implied by commonly used models of female labour supply are: (1) a woman will choose to work if her offered wage exceeds her reservation wage evaluated at zero hours of work, and (2) a woman who works will choose her hours of work so as to equate her reservation wage (evaluated at her actual hours of work) with her offered wage. The implication of the second decision rule for actual behaviour is presumably that working women will look for job situations that allow them to come as close as possible to supplying the amounts of labour that would equate their offered and reservation wage rates. This analytical framework focusses attention on factors that are expected to affect women's offered and reservation wage rates.

The *direct effects* of the time, effort and expense of having and caring for children are usually viewed as affecting a woman's labour supply behaviour via her reservation wage function. The coefficients of child status variables in the equations for the probability of work and for the hours of work are hypothesized to reflect these direct effects. As stated in the Introduction, the problems of estimating the direct effects of children on female labour supply are examined in section 5.

The child bearing and rearing roles of women are also hypothesized to have *indirect effects* on female labour supply via human capital investment effects on women's offered wage rates. Women who have children and who work less during their active child bearing and rearing years will accumulate less on-the-job experience because of their reduced labour supply. Another way in which children are thought to reduce the job-related human capital that women accumulate involves anticipatory behaviour on the part of employers, women's families, and women themselves. The returns to job-related training are realized through working. If most women work less than most men over their lifetimes (presumably because most women have children), then employers and others (including women themselves) may be less willing to make training investments in women because the expected returns are lower than for equally capable men. Economic theory implies a positive relationship between the offered wage rates of individuals and their stocks of job-related human capital.

Suppose that children have negative effects on women's offered wage rates via the effects of children on job-related human capital accumulation. The sign of the resulting *offered wage effects* on female labour supply will determine whether the *indirect child status effects* on female labour supply are positive or negative. This is the motivation for selectively reviewing in section 4 reported estimation results for the responses of the hours of work of married women to changes in their offered wage rates.

12.3. Basic econometric choices

All of the econometric issues to be considered in this section can be discussed within the framework of the static, one-period model. Models of this sort have provided the analytical basis for a large body of applied research on female labour supply. See, for example, Heckman (1974b, 1976a, 1980); Nakamura *et al.* (1979); Nakamura and Nakamura (1981, 1983); and the long list of studies given in Killingsworth (1983, table 4.3, pp. 193-199). This model also forms a helpful point of departure for considering a number of the issues dealt with in later sections of this paper.

The static, one-period model and various extensions of it are discussed more fully in the previous chapter. For convenience, we restate the key equations of the model.

Let H denote a woman's hours of work in a given time period. Her offered wage is denoted by w, and her reservation wage evaluated at her actual hours of work is denoted by $w^*(H)$. Let Z be a vector of personal characteristics affecting productivity in paid work, such as years of schooling, and of variables which characterize labour market conditions, such as the unemployment rate; let Z^* be a vector of predetermined variables affecting the value a woman places on her off-the-job (or nonmarket) time, such as how many children she has; and let Y stand for household income in the given time period excluding the earnings of the woman herself.

Suppose that a woman's *reservation wage* obeys the relationship

$$\ln w^*(H) = \begin{cases} \beta_0 + Z^*\beta_1 + \beta_3 \ln w + \beta_4 H + u^* & \text{if } H > 0 \\ \beta_0 + Z^*\beta_1 + \beta_2 Y + u^* & \text{if } H = 0, \end{cases} \tag{1}$$

and that her *offered wage* is given by

$$\ln w = \alpha_0 + Z\alpha_1 + u. \tag{2}$$

Then the probability the woman will work in the specified time period is given by

$$P(H > 0) = P[\ln w > \ln w^*(0)] = F(\phi), \tag{3}$$

where F denotes a cumulative density function for $(u^* - u)$,

$$\phi = (1/\sigma)[(\alpha_0 - \beta_0) + Z\alpha_1 + Z^*\beta_1 - \beta_2 Y], \tag{4}$$

and σ is the standard deviation of $(u^* - u)$. If a woman who works chooses her hours of work so as to equate her reservation wage evaluated at her actual hours of work with her offered wage, then her hours of work will be given by

$$H = (1/\beta_4)[(1-\beta_3)\ln w - \beta_0 - Z^*\beta_1 - \beta_2 Y - u^*], \qquad (5)$$

In equations (1)-(5), the α's and β's are parameters to be estimated.

12.3.1. Dealing with limited dependent variables

A probability, such as the probability of work in a year, must lie between 0 and 1. Also hours of work must be nonnegative. Thus both the probability of work and hours of work are limited dependent variables. The simplest estimation approaches ignore this aspect of these variables. For example, relationships (3) and (4) for the probability of work can be approximated by a *linear probability model*. A dummy variable set equal to 1 for each woman who works and set equal to 0 otherwise can be regressed on the variables in Z, Z^* and Y. Linear probability models were estimated in many of the earlier micro data studies of female labour supply.

One drawback of the linear probability model is that the predicted values for the probability of work may not fall in the 0-1 interval within which probabilities must lie. A second problem is that the ordinary least squares (OLS) estimates of the standard errors of the coefficient estimates will not be appropriate. Two estimation methods which overcome the first of these problems, and which may yield more appropriate estimated standard errors, are logit and probit analysis. If F in (3) is the standard normal cumulative density function, then *probit analysis* is the estimation method to choose. If F is thought to be the logistic cumulative density function, then *logit analysis* is the proper estimation method.

12.3.2. Sample selection

Available data sources contain no information on many factors believed to affect individual probabilities of work. Moreover some of these factors may also affect women's offered wage rates and hours of work, and may be correlated with some of the included variables in the equations for hours of work and the offered wage. If the hours of work and offered wage equations are estimated using data only for women who work, and without regard for the omitted factors also affecting the selection of who works, the estimated coefficients may be subject to *selection biases*.

There are two econometric approaches to selection bias problems that have been widely used in studies of female labour supply. Both usually presume that F in (3) is the standard normal cumulative density function. The first approach, called *Tobit estimation*, usually involves treating the relationships for the probability of work and the hours equation as an integrated model. This treatment is consistent with the theoretical derivation of the model. In practice, however, the Tobit assumption of an integrated model may be inappropriate because some of the included (or omitted) variables have different types of effects on the decision to work versus the choice of hours of work.

An alternative approach is the two step estimation procedure sometimes called Heckit analysis. In *Heckit analysis*, the parameters of (4) are first estimated using probit analysis. These estimation results are used to compute values for a *selection bias term* defined as

$$\lambda = f(\phi)/F(\phi), \tag{6}$$

where f is the standard normal density function, F is the standard normal cumulative density function, and ϕ denotes the estimated probit index defined in (4). Under certain assumptions, when the Heckit λ is included as an additional regressor in the offered wage and hours equations it will control for selection bias effects, and these equations can be appropriately estimated using only data for women who work. This is important because, in most data sets, wage information is available only for women who work. (For fuller discussion on this topic see Heckman, 1974b, 1976a, 1977, 1980, 1987; and Gronau, 1974. See also Amemiya, 1984; Paarsch, 1984; Nakamura and Nakamura, 1989; and Wales and Woodland, 1980.)

12.3.3. Bias problems associated with specific explanatory variables

The basic cause of coefficient bias problems are correlations between included explanatory variables and omitted factors. Because of these correlations, the coefficient estimates for the included explanatory variables pick up some of the effects of the omitted factors in a proxy sense. Hence these estimated coefficients will not appropriately reflect what the impacts on the dependent variable would be of specified changes in the associated explanatory variables. The selection biases discussed in the previous subsection are due to correlations between explanatory variables in the equation of interest and omitted factors that also affect selection into the group for whom the equation is being estimated.

Another source of correlations that can cause coefficient bias problems are omitted factors which are also determinants of an included explanatory variable in the equation. For example, tastes for a job-oriented versus a home-oriented life style may affect hours of work and may also be determinants of the offered wage variable included in the hours equation via the effects of these tastes on human capital accumulation. (For discussion and references concerning tests for bias problems of this sort see Nakamura and Nakamura, 1981b, 1985c.) There are two approaches which have been commonly adopted for coping with this problem. These approaches can be most easily understood in a specific context.

For example, suppose the wage variable in the hours of work equation (5) is correlated with the equation error term, but that the observable factors in Z (from the offered wage equation) are uncorrelated with the error term for the hours equation. In the one approach, the right-hand side of the offered wage equation (2) is substituted for the wage variable in the hours equation, yielding a *reduced form* hours equation. In the other approach, the parameters of the wage equation are estimated in some appropriate way, and then predicted values for the wage variable are substituted for the actual values in the hours equation. This second approach is called *instrumental variables (IV)* estimation.

12.4. Estimating offered wage effects on female labour supply

Suppose it is true that children tend to reduce the amounts of job-related human capital that women accumulate, and that offered wage rates are an increasing function of job-related human capital. (For discussion and empirical evidence relevant to these assertions, see Corcoran *et al.*, 1983; Cox, 1984; England, 1982, 1984; Jones and Long, 1979; Mincer and Ofek, 1982; Mincer and Polachek, 1974, 1978; Polachek, 1979, 1981; and Sandell and Shapiro, 1978, 1980.) Then *the indirect, offered wage-related effects of children on female labour supply will be negative if there is a positive relationship between women's labour supply and their offered wage rates.*

A woman's expected *unconditional labour* supply can be factored into the *probability of work* in a given period (that is, the probability of positive hours of work) times the *expected hours of work conditional on the decision to work.* This suggests that estimates of offered wage effects on the probability of work and on the hours of work for women who work can be obtained from the estimated coefficients of a wage variable in equations for the probability of work and for the hours of work for those who do.

The hours equation (5) contains the offered wage variable ln w.

In the index for the probability of work (4), the right-hand side of the offered wage equation (2) has been substituted for ln w. The reason for this substitution is that offered wage values are not usually available for those who did not work. The variables included in the index for the probability of work need to be ones that can be observed for women who did not work as well as for those who did.

In (4), Z^* is a vector of variables believed to affect women's reservation wage rates, while Z appears because the right-hand side of (2) has been substituted for ln w. If there are variables in Z which are not included in Z^*, then the response of the probability of work to women's offered wage rates might be inferred from the estimated coefficients of these variables. However, it is difficult to think of variables which would affect what employers would be willing to pay women and that would definitely not affect their reservation wage rates. For this and other reasons, efforts to estimate offered wage effects on female labour supply have focussed primarily on the hours equation.

12.4.1. Wage effects on the hours of work for working women

Many authors still seem convinced that the available empirical evidence shows that working women (or, at least, working wives) tend to increase their hours of work in response to increases in their wage rates. For instance, Blau and Ferber write:

> "With respect to the hours decision, empirical evidence indicates that for men ... they do not decrease, or may even increase, the amount of nonmarket time as their wage rate goes up. ... The situation is quite different for women ... empirical studies for the most part find that women's labor supply is strongly positively related to the wage rate." (Blau and Ferber, 1986, p. 95).

Nevertheless, estimates for married women of the impact of a wage change on hours of work that are small and sometimes negative have been obtained in a number of studies based on cross-sectional and panel micro data. Using micro data from the 1971 Census of Canada, Nakamura *et al.* (1979, p. 800) obtain estimates of the wage response of hours of work for married women in the prime working age groups of 20-24, 25-49, and so on through 45-49 that are in the same range as the responses reported by other researchers for prime age men. Of course, Canadian and U.S. wives might differ in their work behaviour because of a variety of country-specific factors. For instance, U.S. couples typically file joint tax returns while Canadian wives who work are taxed as separate individuals just like their husbands. These concerns are addressed and dismissed in Nakamura and Nakamura (1981a). The tax-corrected estimation results reported in that paper are based on micro data from the 1970 U.S. Census and from the 1971 Census of Canada.

Other researchers have suggested that perhaps wives working full-time might exhibit wage responses similar to those of men, but that wives working part-time would exhibit the large positive elasticities that some have argued should be expected for working women. In Nakamura and Nakamura (1983, p. 246), estimates of the wage response for hours of work are presented separately for U.S. and Canadian wives in five different child status categories and in the two hours-of-work categories of part-time (less than 1,400 in the year) and full-time (1,400 hours or more). The estimated elasticities for women working part-time are found to be similar to those for women working full-time.

Killingsworth (1983, pp. 200-201) has suggested still another reason why the results presented in Nakamura *et al.* (1979) and in Nakamura and Nakamura (1981) may be aberrant. He points out that years of work experience are not directly controlled for in these studies, and also that a child status variable is included as a proxy for experience in the log wage equations. These conjectures are explored empirically in Nakamura and Nakamura (1985b, pp. 180-190 and pp. 278-293). The results are in line with those reported in Nakamura *et al.* (1979) and in Nakamura and Nakamura (1981a).

By now, a number of other researchers have also reported offered wage effects on the hours of work of working women that are small in magnitude, and sometimes negative, as for men. Studies reporting results of this sort include Robinson and Tomes (1985), Stelcner and Breslaw (1985), Smith and Stelcner (1988), and Mroz (1987).

On the basis of these results, *we conclude that probably the wage responses of hours of work for married women are modest, as for men*, and possibly negative. This conclusion is further supported by similar estimates from studies based on negative income tax experimental data for men and for women (Killingsworth, 1983, pp. 398-399, table 6.2). This means that, except for impacts of women's child bearing and rearing activities on their wage rates that are relatively large, *the indirect effects of children on the hours of work of working women that are transmitted via impacts on their wage rates are probably not of great importance.*

This does not mean, however, that the indirect, offered wage effects of children on the probability of work are small.

12.4.2. Wage effects on the probability of work

Economic theory implies that when a woman's offered wage rises this will increase the opportunity cost of her nonmarket time and will provide an incentive for her to substitute more hours of work for nonwork time. Also, however, for a working woman a wage increase means (by definition) that she will earn more even without changing her hours of work, and economic theory implies that a higher income will lead her to increase her consumption of desirable "goods" including time off the job. In other words, economic theory implies that for those who work the *positive substitution effects* of a wage change on the hours of work will be counterbalanced to some (theoretically undetermined) extent by *negative income effects*. Even a negative net relationship between women's offered wage rates and the hours of work for those who work cannot be ruled out on theoretical grounds.

With regard to the decision to work (as opposed to the choice of hours of work) there should only be positive substitution effects of a wage change on the decision to work, since a change in the offered wage does not change the earned income of a women who is not working. The lack of a strong positive relationship between the offered wage rates and the hours of work *of working women* cannot be interpreted as evidence against this theoretical implication. (A fuller discussion of substitution and income effects is provided in chapter 11).

12.5. Estimating the direct effects of children on female labour supply

Whether or not children have important indirect effects on female labour supply, available empirical evidence suggests that some of the direct effects of children are negative and possibly large. Consensus concerning the magnitudes of these direct effects of children awaits consensus concerning the proper methodology for estimating them.

12.5.1. Alternative estimates presented by Schultz

Schultz (1978) compares estimates of the labour supply responses to the number of children ever born for several of the estimation methods discussed in section 3. In table 1 we present some of his results in elasticity form, as Schultz presents these results. An elasticity gives the percentage change in the dependent variable in response to a one percent change in the designated explanatory variable. Schultz's *OLS results for all women* (with hours of work at zero for those who did not work) are shown in column 1 in the top panel of table 1. Schultz's *Tobit estimates* of these same labour supply responses are presented in column 2. The Tobit approach, which also uses data for all women, allows for the limited nature of the dependent variable (hours of work cannot be negative), for the fact that wages cannot be observed for those who do not work, and for the possibility of selection bias problems. Compared in terms of their magnitudes, the estimates in columns 1 and 2 are quite similar. Both sets of estimates imply there is a strong negative relationship between the expected labour supply of a woman and the number of children she has. These estimates are consistent with the popular belief that a female employee who has a baby is likely to quit or to drastically reduce her hours of work.

Schultz's estimates shown in column 3 of table 1 are for the same linear hours equation for which estimation results are shown in column 1, except that now the *OLS estimates* of the response parameters are computed using data *for only those women who worked* (that is, for women with positive hours of work). No correction has been made for possible selection bias problems, but it has been established elsewhere that, in this context, allowing for selection bias may not greatly change the estimated child status responses (see Nakamura and Nakamura 1985b, section 4.3.5). The estimated responses shown in column 3 are small in magnitude compared to the results when data for all women are used (columns 1 and 2).

Table 1. Estimates of elasticity of annual labour supply of wives
with respect to children ever born

| | Annual hours of work | | | Probability of work |
| | All wives | | Wives who worked | All wives |
	OLS	ML Tobit	OLS	Logit
White, 18-24	-.55	-.76	-.10	-.60
White, 25-29	-1.04	-1.12	-.29	-.80
White, 30-34	-.51	-.62	.06	-.49
White, 35-39	-.47	-.51	-.18	-.33
	Instrumental variable for children ever born			
White, 18-24	-.24	-.39	.05	-.37
White, 25-49	-.95	-.90	-.14	-.74
White, 30-34	-.92	-1.13	.07	-.95
White, 35-39	-1.13	-1.41	-.27	-1.06

Source: Schultz (1978), p. 299, table 6.

In column 4 of table 1 we show Schultz's logit analysis estimates of the elasticity of female labour supply with respect to the children ever born. A woman's unconditional expected labour supply in a year can be represented as the product of the probability she will work sometime during the year times her expected hours of work if she does work. The elasticity estimates in column 4 only take account of child status effects on the first of these two components into which unconditional expected labour supply can be factored, while the elasticity estimates in column 3 can be thought of as measures of the importance of the second of these components. The elasticity estimates in column 4 for the probability of work are almost as large in magnitude as the estimates in column 1 and in column 2 for the unconditional annual labour supply responses to children born.

A first implication of the results in the top panel of table 1 is that *child-related variations in labour supply primarily manifest themselves in alterations in the propensity to work.* This is not a new observation. In 1969, Bowen and Finegan wrote that "variations in hours worked [for working wives] associated with the presence of children of various ages are so much smaller than the variations in participation that the set of full-time-equivalent rates [for the labour supply of all married women] is dominated by the relationships between the children variables and the adjusted participation rates" (p. 100).

A second implication is that *it may not be appropriate to model the decision to work and the choice of hours of work as aspects of a common underlying behavioural response process*. Schultz (1978, pp. 297-298) observes, "it might be argued that the two choices, first of entering the market labor force and then of determining how many hours to work in the market, arise in different ways, or at least that some variables would receive different weights in the two decisions such as fixed costs of entering the labor force." On the basis of a more recent analysis of alternative models and estimation methods, Mroz (1987, p. 790) also concludes, "the hours of work decisions made when the woman is in the labor force appear quite distinct from her labor force participation decision." (This is not a new finding. See, for example, Lewis, 1967 and Ben Porath, 1973. Despite this, however, the Tobit specification of an integrated model for the decision to work and for hours of work has enjoyed considerable popularity in recent years.) As in the Schultz study, Mroz finds that the Tobit estimates of child-related labour supply responses, obtained using the data for all women, are much larger than the estimates obtained using only data for women who worked.

12.5.2. More on instrumental child status variables

Schultz and others argue that the child bearing behaviour and the labour supply of women are determined by some of the same variables. That is, "fertility may be appropriately viewed in the long run as an endogenous choice variable that is jointly and simultaneously determined by a couple in conjunction with the wife's decision as to how much time she will allocate to the market labor force over her married lifetime (Schultz, 1978, p. 283)". Following Schultz's lead, a number of other researchers have estimated models of female labour supply in which fertility decisions are treated as "endogenous". For instance, in describing his study based on a complex model of female labour supply and fertility, Moffitt (1984b, pp. 263-265) writes that

"... labour supply and fertility decisions are modelled as completely joint in the same sense as the consumption of two goods is joint. ... The implication of these considerations for econometric estimation is primarily that only exogenous variables should be included in the fertility and female labour-supply equations."

If fertility decisions are endogenous in this sense, one implication is that child-status variables contained in Z^* may be correlated with the error term u^* in the hours equation (5). In this case it may be appropriate to deal with the endogeneity of the child status variables by using an *instrumental variables* (IV) estimation method.

An IV method involves replacing the original child status variables appearing in the labour supply equations by estimated linear combinations of "exogenous" variables. Thus the child status variables are split into "explained" and "unexplained" portions, and the unexplained portions of the original child status variables are relegated to the equation disturbance terms. The hope is that the explained portions of the child status variables (the linear combinations of exogenous variables) will be uncorrelated with the omitted, persistent tastes and preconditions affecting both child status and labour supply, and hence will not serve as proxies for these omitted factors.

The elasticity estimates presented in the bottom panel of table 1 correspond, column by column, to those in the top panel, except that they are computed from the coefficient estimates for an instrumental variable for the number of children born. Compared with the elasticity estimates in the top panel, these estimates are consistently less negative for wives younger than 30, but are almost always more negative for wives 30 and older. These differences are small in magnitude when only data for working wives are used (column 3) and tend to be quite large when data for all wives are used (columns 1, 2 and 4). The figures in columns 1, 2 and 4 of the bottom panel suggest, for instance, that a married woman who has been working will be likely to quit if she has a child when she is over 30.

The elasticity estimates in the bottom panel of table 1 might be questioned, however. Even though the motivation for using an instrumental child status variable is clear, it is not clear that the approach solves the underlying correlation (or endogeneity) problem. The difficulty lies with the near impossibility of finding suitable variables to use as instruments for the child status variables. With respect to Schultz's own choice of instrumental variables in his 1978 study, he writes:

"I will assume here that the wife's residential origins at age 16, her age, and the schooling of both spouses are exogenous determinants

of fertility, but that these variables exert no direct role in
determining the current labor market behavior of the wife. Rural,
farm, and Southern origins are frequently stressed in the demographic
literature as correlates of U.S. fertility. The wife's age is
strongly related to children-ever-born, at least through age 40, and
is hardly related to labor force behavior within the narrow age
subsamples examined here (18-24, and then 5-year age brackets from
ages 25-64). It should be repeated, however, that there is no strong
theoretical presumption that these identifying restrictions are in
some sense 'correct', but they are proposed only as a starting
point." (Schultz, 1978, p. 291)

Unfortunately, it seems conceivable that a woman's residential origins, and
her own and her spouse's schooling experiences, could shape her views about
both child bearing and the benefits and suitability of mothers working. Hence,
an instrumental child status variable based on these residential origins and
schooling variables may still pick up both direct effects of children on a
woman's labour supply behavior and the effects of taste factors affecting her
fertility and also her labour supply. Certainly these "exogenous" variables
will not reflect any of the truly chance variation in fertility due to factors
like contraceptive failure or multiple births. In fact, it could be that
variables like residential origins and years of schooling almost exclusively
reflect the variability over women in child status that is due to persistent
tastes for home-oriented versus job-oriented activities. Thus the taste-related
proxy effects associated with instrumental child status variables could be
stronger, rather than weaker as hoped, than the proxy effects associated with
child status variables that are directly entered into female labour supply
equations.

Moreover, even if suitable exogenous variables could be found to serve
as instruments for a single child status variable such as the number of
children born, the limited availability of suitable exogenous variables and
the limited understanding of the determinants of various aspects of fertility
behaviour must surely mean that very few dimensions of a woman's child status
can be dealt with using an instrumental variables approach. (For an introduction to some of the aspects of a woman's child status that might be of
importance, see, for example, Heckman *et al.*, 1985; Hill and Stafford, 1985b).
In Schultz's 1978 study, the only child status variable is a linear term for
the number of children ever born. The following passage makes it clear that
Schultz recognizes this shortcoming of an instrumental variables approach:

"But unfortunately, the framework used by economists to interpret differences in fertility (or surviving numbers of children) says little about the factors affecting the timing and spacing of child-bearing. It may not be the number of children a woman has borne, or expects to bear, that directly affects her current labor supply, but rather the current presence of preschool-aged children in the household or the age of the youngest child. ... There is also evidence that the direct association between numbers of children and the wife's labor supply is nonlinear, with the first child having by far the greatest effect." (Schultz, 1978, p. 286).

12.5.3. A fertility control-related instrumental variables approach

In the search for a better set of exogenous variables to use as instruments for child status variables, Rosenzweig and Schultz (1985) take a closer look at the production process for babies:

"Unlike the consumption by households of television sets or food, the level of fertility is determined by the allocation of resources to limit the biologically determined production of birth-fertility supply. Given that such control is costly and imperfect, and the biological capacity to bear children (fecundity) is stochastic and mostly unaffected by choice behavior, the number of children born to a couple (society) may not exactly correspond to either the couple's (societal) expectations of or preferences for (given costless control) its family (population) size. Moreover, an individual couple may learn about its own specific supply constraints over time ..." (Rosenzweig and Schultz, 1985, p. 992).

The actual number of births to a couple in a given time period is modelled as a sum of a time invariant, couple-specific fecundity factor; a random component; an age factor; and fertility control measures.

The *fecundity factor* is found to be associated with persistent differences in labour supply. Rosenzweig and Schultz write:

"The estimates indicate that among couples whose fecundity is one standard deviation above the population mean, the proportion of months between 1973 and 1975 in which the wife participated in the labor market was reduced by 16 percent. As was evident for fertility and contraception, moreover, the effects of fecundity variation appear to increase over the life cycle-among the highly fecund couples, the probability that the wife participated in the labor market was 12 percent lower in 1973 and was 17 percent lower in 1975." (Rosenzweig and Schultz, 1985, pp. 1009-1010).

In contrast to these persistent fecundity effects, Rosenzweig and Schultz find that unexpected births (that is, the *random component* of fertility) affect the timing of a woman's labour supply but have little or no effect on the amount of labour a woman supplies over her lifetime. Rosenzweig and Schultz report:

> "With respect to quantitative effects, the associations between actual fertility in the 1970-72 period and the wife's participation in 1973 and 1975 overstate both the immediate (1973) negative and longer-term labor supply responses to an unanticipated birth. The wife's probability of labor force participation is reduced at the sample means by 40 percent in 1973, and by 28 percent in 1975, in response to an actual birth between 1970-72. The arrival of an *unanticipated* birth in the same 30-month period (less 9 months for the pregnancy) ... would reduce the wife's likelihood of participation by only 18 percent in the following year (1973), and *increases* the participation probability by 14 percent in 1975." (Rosenzweig and Schultz, 1985, p. 1011).

For a better understanding of the Rosenzweig-Schultz results, it is important to take a closer look at their estimation methodology. They estimate a *reproduction technology function*, with a measure of actual fertility as the dependent variable. The explanatory variables are several variables for the type and amount of birth control used, births before 1970, coital frequency, whether the woman smoked, and the woman's age and age squared. However, all of these variables are treated as endogenous (and hence potentially correlated with the equation error term) except age and age squared. Taking an 4 approach, estimated linear combinations of variables that are asserted to be exogenous are substituted for the explanatory variables other than age and age squared. The so-called *exogenous variables* are personal characteristics including age, education, religious background and the husband's income, as well as a number of area-specific characteristics such as city size and the per-capita number of obstetrician-gynecologists. The difference between the actual birth rate of couple j in period i (n_{ij}) and the predicted birth rate based on the estimated reproduction technology function (n^e_{ij}) is assumed to be the sum of the couple-specific fecundity factor and the random component. In particular, the *fecundity factor* for each couple is computed as

$$\mu_j = \sum_{i=1}^{t} (n_{ij} - n^e_{ij})/t$$

where t is the number of time periods, and the *random component* for each
couple in each time period is given by

$$\varepsilon_{ij} = n_{ij} - n^e_{ij} - \mu_j.$$

Notice first of all that the predicted birth rate variable, n^e_{ij}, obtained
from the reproduction technology function is similar (though more sophisticated) in its makeup to the instrumental child status variable in Schultz's
1978 study (see the discussion of this study in the previous subsection). In
Schultz's 1978 study the instrumental child status variable is a function of
variables such as the wife's age, education, and place of origin. In the
Rosenzweig-Schultz study, the predicted birth rate is modelled as a function
of the wife's age and a number of other variables for factors such as contraceptive choice and usage; but the factors other than age are in turn represented as functions of background factors for each woman, including her age
and education. In Schultz's 1978 study he views the instrumental child status
variable as *independent* of tastes and preferences which might also affect work
behaviour, while in the Rosenzweig-Schultz study it is argued that n^e_{ij} *captures*
these same tastes and preferences. As should be clear from our concluding
remarks in the previous subsection, we find the line of argument in the
Rosenzweig-Schultz study more persuasive.

A second point is that the couple-specific fecundity factor and the
random component are determined as the residual difference between the actual
and the predicted birth rate. Hence any persistent taste or learning effects
on the actual birth rate of a couple that are not captured by the predicted
birth rate will end up as part of the fecundity factor or the random component.
For example, previous work experience is not controlled for in the values of
n^e_{ij}. Starting to work may reduce a woman's desired family size and lead to
greater use of birth control. But this will not necessarily be captured by the
instrumental fertility control variables which do not depend on past work
experience, and hence this effect may show up as a lower value for the
fecundity factor or for the random component.

12.5.4. An experimental approach

Rosenzweig and Wolpin (1980) suggest another innovative approach to the problem
of obtaining measures of child status impacts on female labour supply that are

not confounded with the effects of general tastes and preconditions. Rosenzweig and Wolpin claim:

"In particular, we show how a natural event, the occurrence of a multiple birth or 'twins', can be used as an instrument for exogenous fertility movements. The variable we propose, a twins outcome in the first birth, approximates the social experiment we wish to perform not only in that some families receive an unanticipated child, while others do not, but also in that the treatment and control groups are randomly selected with respect to characteristics that may be related to market participation. It is therefore unnecessary to utilize any information on the determinants of labor supply behavior in order to determine the 'true' exogenous fertility effect by this method." (Rosenzweig and Wolpin, 1980, pp. 335-336).

They go on to explain:

"To see why the occurrence of twins in the first pregnancy, 'twins first', leads to the appropriate experiment, consider, instead, a comparison of women who have had twins in any birth and women who have not. ... It is obvious that women with more births - and thus women with, on average, greater desired fertility - will be over-represented in the sample of twins families. The labor supply of women with twins will therefore reflect in part any relationship between unobserved tastes for children and/or tastes for home time. ... Moreover, the per pregnancy probability of twins appears to rise with parity. ... The first birth has the desirable feature that the population of women who experience twins in that birth would prefer the same completed family size as women who do not experience twins in the first birth ..." (Rosenzweig and Wolpin, 1980, p. 336).

Rosenzweig and Wolpin find that an "extra" child on the first birth (before age 35) reduces the mother's current probability of labour force participation by 35 percentage points for women 15-24 years of age, and by about 10 percentage points for women 25-34 years of age.

In the Rosenzweig-Wolpin study, data are pooled from two national random surveys of women: a 1965 survey conducted by the Office of Population Research and a 1973 survey carried out by the U.S. Department of Health, Education and Welfare. Of 15,000 available observations for women 15-44 years of age, 12,605 are used. The main reason for excluding observations is childlessness. The twins-first methodology requires a data sample for women who have had at least one birth. The necessity of excluding childless women is a drawback of the methodology. There may be a fairly strong association between having even one child and a preference for a home-oriented rather than a career-orientated life style.

Of the 12,605 observations, 87 were for women whose first children were twins. The rarity of multiple births is another drawback of the twins-first methodology.

A third difficulty from the perspective of this paper is the Rosenzweig-Wolpin focus on "exogenous fertility movements". The labour supply responses of women to planned children - which is what most children are - may be quite different from their responses to accidental extra children - which is what an "extra" twin is. There may also be scale or threshold effects associated with the care of babies.

We have reluctantly come to the conclusion that, despite its experimental appeal, the Rosenzweig-Wolpin twins-first approach is not a practical methodology for estimating child-related effects on female labour supply. However, a careful consideration of this study has greatly enhanced our own understanding of the basic purposes of and problems with estimating these effects.

12.5.5. Unobservable fixed effects

Bias problems in estimating the coefficients of child status variables in labour supply equations result from correlations between unmeasured tastes and preconditions affecting both labour supply and child status. As already noted, the IV solution to bias problems involves partitioning the child status variables into "explained" and "unexplained" portions, and moving the unexplained portions to the error terms of the reformulated labour supply equations. An alternative approach is to attempt instead to remove the offending unobservables from the error terms of the original labour supply equations.

Heckman and MaCurdy (1980, 1982) present a life cycle model of female labour supply in which intertemporal factors affect current labour supply only through an individual-specific term which is the Lagrange multiplier associated with the lifetime budget constraint. Under certain assumptions, this individual-specific term can be treated as fixed over time for each individual. If an estimation method is used which effectively accounts for or eliminates this individual fixed effects term, two important implications follow for the coefficient estimates of the child status variables in a model of current labour supply. First, the coefficients of the child status variables can be interpreted as reflecting only the current direct impacts of children on a woman's labour supply. Second, one might hope that persistent, individual-specific factors, that may be correlated with child status, like tastes for a home-oriented life style, will be accounted for, and hence will not result in biased estimates of the current period, direct child status effects due to spurious correlations.

12.5.6. Unobservable effects which are persistent but not fixed over time

Unobservable factors which persist over time, but are not fixed, cannot be eliminated by first differencing or by using other fixed effects estimation methods. However, in some cases it may be possible to deliberately introduce proxy variables to account for these effects. Unobservable factors which are not left in the disturbance terms of the labour supply equations cannot be picked up (unintentionally) in a proxy sense by the child status variables.

Nakamura and Nakamura argue that if there are important unobservable factors which affect the labour supply of a woman year after year, then the effects of these unobservable factors will be embedded in the observable past work behaviour of the woman. In this case, it should be possible to at least partially remove these taste factors from the disturbance terms of the labour supply relationships by introducing some measure of past labour supply into the relationships to be estimated. This is the motivation for the Inertia Model of female labour supply developed in Nakamura and Nakamura (1985b). In the empirical implementation of this model, the variables used as proxies for unobservable preconditions and tastes for work are the observed employment status (worked or did not work) in the previous year, and the hours of work and wage rate in the previous year for those who worked then. In the Inertia Model, labour supply behaviour is found to be persistent in the sense that women who work (do not work) in one year are more likely to continue working (not working) in the next year even after accounting for the effects of all of the variables that have customarily been included in models of female labour supply. This persistence is so strong, in fact, that even women who have just had a baby are found to be likely to continue working if they worked a substantial number of hours in the previous year.

Other studies in which recent work behaviour is taken into account have yielded weak estimated child status responses like those reported by Nakamura and Nakamura. Johnson and Pencavel (1984) and Jones and Long (1980) estimated

models of female labour supply controlling for labour supply in the previous
year and obtained estimated child status effects which are small in magnitude.
Based on a multinomial logit analysis of National Longitudinal Survey (NLS)
data, Shaw (1983, p. 49) finds that "even with children present, once the woman
had a history of continuous work, family considerations ... did not cause them
to work less." Picot (1987) obtains similar results for Canadian women using
data from Statistics Canada's Family History Survey. Even (1987) obtains
empirical results confirming this finding in a hazard model of career interruptions following childbirth estimated using data from the 1973 National Survey
of Family Growth. Even (1987, p. 273) finds that "remaining employed late into
pregnancy is a very strong indicator of postchildbirth employment decisions."
Further results indicating that child-related effects on market-work productivity are modest for at least some working women can be found in Cole and
Zuckerman's (1987) case study of the research performance of women in science.

Like the age, residential origins and education variables sometimes used
in computing instrumental child status variables, information on a woman's
employment status and work behaviour in the previous year is readily (and
ethically) available to both researchers and employers. (Nakamura and Nakamura,
1985a, point out that this information could even be cheaply collected on a
recall basis in cross-sectional surveys like the U.S. Census of Population.)
Unlike strictly cross-sectional labour supply equations (with or without
instrumental child status variables), labour supply equations incorporating
variables for work behavior in the previous year explain a large portion of
the observed variability over time in the labour supply of individual women
(see Nakamura and Nakamura, 1985b). The higher this predictive ability is for
a model of labour supply behaviour, the less room there is for systematic
"mistakes" in prediction that are the essence of statistical discrimination.
Statistical discrimination results precisely when some individuals do not
behave (or would not have behaved if given the chance) as is predicted by the
(formal or informal) behavioural model which is used for selecting the individuals who will receive desired benefits or opportunities. Another advantage
of the estimation approach advocated in Nakamura and Nakamura (1985b) is that
it can be adapted relatively easily to allow for differences in child-related
labour supply responses associated with characteristics of the mother, the
children, or the mother's job or profession.

12.6. Concluding remarks

In this paper, direct and indirect child-related effects on female labour supply are distinguished. The direct effects are associated with changes in women's reservation wage rates, while the indirect effects are conceptualized as operating through the impacts of decisions about human capital accumulation on women's offered wage rates. Basic econometric choices are reviewed concerning the limited nature of the dependent variables in models of female labour supply, sample selection problems, and bias problems associated with specific explanatory variables.

There is considerable controversy in the literature concerning the magnitudes of various child-related effects on women's wage rates. However, both economic theory and available empirical results suggest that women's child bearing and rearing roles are responsible, to some degree, for the apparent wage disadvantage of working women versus working men. If this is so, then the indirect, offered wage-related effects of children on female labour supply will be negative if there is a positive relationship between women's labour supply and their offered wage rates, and positive otherwise. Studies of these wage effects on female labour supply are selectively reviewed in section 4. We conclude that the wage responses of hours of work for working married women are modest, as for men, and possibly negative. This suggests that the indirect effects of children on the hours of work of working women (as opposed to the probability of work) are probably modest. We note that little is known about the importance of indirect child-related effects on the probability of work, largely because information on wage offers is usually available only for those who work.

The rest of the paper deals with the estimation of the direct effects of children on female labour supply. On the basis of comparative estimation results presented by Schultz, we find that direct child-related effects on the probability of work are quantitatively more important than on the hours of work for women who do work. We also side with Schultz and Mroz in concluding that it is important to estimate separate relationships for the probability of work, and for hours of work for women who do work.

Much of the disagreement concerning the magnitude of direct child-related effects on female labour supply is rooted in potential bias problems due to correlations between factors omitted from the labour supply relationships and the included child status variables. Two basic approaches to this problem are discussed.

The instrumental variables (IV) approach involves trying to purge the child status variable(s) of those components correlated with the true error(s) term for the labour supply relationship(s). Studies taking this approach by Schultz (1978) and Rosenzweig and Schultz (1985) are discussed in some detail. An experimentally oriented approach due to Rosenzweig and Wolpin (1980) is also reviewed.

The other approach to dealing with coefficient bias problems is to try to remove from the error term(s) of the labour supply relationship(s) the components that are correlated with the included child status variables. Methodologies which could accomplish this purpose by Heckman and MaCurdy (1980, 1982) and by Nakamura and Nakamura (1985b) are briefly discussed.

Our hope is that this review article will help to clarify basic issues concerning the estimation of child-related effects on female labour supply. In turn, we hope this will encourage further and more fruitful empirical studies on this important research topic.

HOW ECONOMICS, PSYCHOLOGY, AND SOCIOLOGY MIGHT PRODUCE
A UNIFIED THEORY OF FERTILITY AND LABOUR FORCE PARTICIPATION[1]

Boone A. Turchi
Department of Economics and Carolina Population Center
The University of North Carolina at Chapel Hill
CB # 3305, Gardner Hall
CHAPEL HILL, NC 27599
U.S.A.

13.1. Introduction

As a result of the sharp declines of the past two decades, aggregate fertility rates in many industrial countries are so low that the twenty-first century will bring negative rates of population growth to those nations of the kind already experienced by, for example, the Federal Republic of Germany. Along with this fertility decline has come a marked increase in labour force participation by married women, especially those with children. In the United States, for example, the labour force participation rate for married women with children under age six rose from 11.9 per cent in 1950 to 49.9 per cent in 1983. Women with school-age children increased their participation rate over the same period from 28.3 per cent to 63.8 per cent (Lehrer and Nerlove, 1986, p. 201).

It would appear that these two trends should be intimately related; however, the causal relationships between fertility and married women's labour force participation remain poorly understood. Many cross-sectional studies of sample survey data have shown that *current family size and structure* and labour force participation are strongly and negatively related, and many researchers have tried to demonstrate that these cross-section associations can be interpreted in causal terms.[2] However, the association of *past* fertility behaviour with *current* labour force participation offers at best only a partial insight into the fertility-labour force participation nexus. The importance of these two behaviours has made them popular objects of study in a number of disciplines including economics, sociology, and psychology, but the research has generally retained its narrow disciplinary focus. A totally successful

---

[1] Thanks to David Claris for producing one of the figures, Lynn Igoe for checking references and Cheryl Ward for updating reference data base.
[2] See Cramer (1980) for a careful analysis of the fertility-labour force participation relationship in the sociological literature.

integration of the insights and emphases of the various disciplines has yet to emerge.

This essay presents a theoretical framework for the analysis of fertility and labour force participation that allows the rigorous and consistent incorporation of insights from a diversity of disciplinary viewpoints. It capitalizes on the fact that both fertility and labour force participation are behaviours that are demonstrably the result of purposeful decision making, and it organizes the framework around an explicit decision theoretic model which serves as the core of the analysis. Use of the constrained utility maximization model to analyse the fertility-labour force participation relationship is certainly not new among economists.[3] What is new here is the attempt to bring sociological and psychological analyses systematically into the utility maximization framework in order to generalize and unify the study of fertility and labour force participation.

The fertility-labour force participation relationship brings many difficulties for the analyst, primarily because it embodies a complex mix of long- and short-run goals and behaviours. Actions today may be designed to bring benefits today or they may be part of a plan that may take two or three decades to complete. In particular, because parenthood is a long-range commitment that requires time (i.e., the sequential arrival and rearing of children) to achieve, an analysis of fertility and labour force participation in the short run must be placed in the context of longer range family size goals. Consequently, this analysis treats the fertility-labour force participation relationship as a special case of the more general demand for children.

Although the micro-economic analysis of fertility dates at least from Gary Becker's seminal piece (1960), many critics of the approach still exist, not least among non-economists. Therefore, the next section provides a brief summary of the criticisms that accompany the use of micro-economic theory to study reproductive behaviour. This review also highlights the areas in which a truly interdisciplinary synthesis can make contributions.

Section 3 sketches a static, long-run, individual-level micro-economic theory of the demand for children. This model provides the framework that allows normative, psychological, and economic influences to interact in determining target family size. Beginning from the traditional individual-level

---

[3] Lehrer and Nerlove (1986) provide a comprehensive review of much of the economics literature and some of the sociological literature.

theoretical perspective, we expand the narrow micro model into a fully-fledged interdisciplinary model by showing how norms and preferences, the subject matter of sociology and psychology, can easily be incorporated into the basic model.

Finally, section 4 addresses one aspect of the fertility-labour force participation relationship by outlining a short-run, sequential model that is contingent upon long-range fertility goals. Fertility and labour force participation can be characterized as an exclusively short-range relationship or as a life-cycle plan or as a mixed set of long-term objectives and short-run sequential behaviour. The approach taken here chooses the latter as a basis for analysis.

13.2. Critiques of the micro-economic approach to reproductive behaviour

In the thirty years since publication of Gary Becker's (1960) application of micro-economic theory to fertility,[4] its role in the analysis of reproductive behaviour has grown steadily. The initial rationale for the use of micro-economic models has remained valid: human reproductive behaviour involves conscious choice in order to keep family size below the biological maximum, it involves significant resource allocation commitments by parents, and it is potentially very much subject to the influence of changing economic conditions.

While the micro-economic fertility literature has grown quite large, it has not convinced skeptics of the ultimate benefit of the approach. Criticisms range from the suitability of the basic assumptions underlying the model to the empirical implementations and, ultimately, the generality and relevance of its insights.[5]

13.2.1. Rationality

Many critics, among them a number of economists, argue that the standard assumption of consistent rational behaviour on the part of husbands and wives

---

[4] Leibenstein (1957) is another early and significant contributor to the economic analysis of fertility.

[5] Thornton and Kim (1980), for example, argue that while people pay lip service to the importance of financial considerations in fertility decision making, few actually make reproductive decisions based upon them.

cannot be supported. Herbert Simon (1978) suggests that the standard rationality assumptions of micro-economic theory can be relaxed with little loss.
Leibenstein (1979) believes that the neoclassical optimization postulate is
inappropriate for fertility analysis and he proposes the *notion of selective
rationality* as an alternative. Supporting that view is Kiser (1979) who cites
results from his own research suggesting that rational choice is exhibited by
only a small proportion of married couples. Other critics suggest that, while
couples may act rationally, micro-economic theory postulates an incorrect
preference structure governing their decisions. Both Namboodiri (1979, p. 292)
and Canlas (1981) argue that wants are governed by a hierarchy of needs that
must be represented by vector-valued utility functions exhibiting lexicographic
preference orderings.

While these objections to consumer theory's rationality assumption have
their force, they are not decisive. As Boland (1981) argues, it is futile to
criticize the neoclassical maximization hypothesis either on logical or
empirical grounds. The maximization hypothesis, he argues, serves as a meta-
physical basis for neoclassical analysis of problems:

> "The research program of neoclassical economics is the challenge of
> finding a neoclassical explanation for any given phenomenon - that
> is, whether it is possible to show that the phenomenon can be seen
> as a logical consequence of maximizing behavior - thus, maximization
> is beyond question for the purpose of accepting the challenge ...
> Since maximization is part of the metaphysics, neoclassical theorists
> too often employ ad hoc methodology in order to deflect possible
> criticism; thus any criticism or defence of neoclassical maximization
> must deal with neoclassical methodology rather than the truth of the
> assumption ... There is nothing intrinsically wrong with the maximi-
> zation hypothesis. The only problem, if there is a problem, resides
> in the methodological attitude of most neoclassical economists. "
> (Boland, 1981, pp. 1035-1036).

More widespread is the view that it is not sufficient simply to model the
preconditions and the outcomes of decisions in order to explain reproductive
behaviour. Rather, it is fundamentally important to model the dynamics of
decision making in order to assess the degree of rationality of the process
itself (Bagozzi and Van Loo, 1978a, 1979; Leibenstein, 1980). Scanzoni (1979)
criticizes the "outcome rationality" of the micro-economic analyses for failing
to study the dynamics of husband/wife negotiating processes in determining
fertility outcomes. Implicit in these views is the notion that decision-making
processes themselves influence the outcomes. If the process were neutral with

respect to the relationship between causes and outcomes then identical sets of causal factors ought to lead to similar outcomes, no matter how decisions are reached (Turchi, 1979).

There is considerable merit to the view that reproductive decision processes are worthy of more careful study (Turchi, 1975, pp. 26-27). However, the decision process may be non-neutral with respect to outcomes without necessarily invalidating the "outcome rationality" approach of consumer theory. If, for example, decision processes do affect outcomes, but they do so randomly and independently of the other factors that determine those outcomes, then the rationality assumption may still be fruitfully used in empirical research (Turchi, 1979, p. 294). Ultimately this issue is empirical, and the results to date do not support the abandonment of the rationality assumptions of the micro-economic models.

13.2.2. Statics versus dynamics

Most couples in the United States reach their completed family size well before the onset of biological subfecundity, and this fact has justified the use of static models in many economic analyses of fertility. Static models assume that decision makers' preferences are constant over the reproductive life cycle and that the factors that determine decisions are likewise constant. The decision problem to be modelled is, then, the determination of long-term equilibrium family size.

There are a number of objections to this approach. Children must be acquired sequentially over time, and there is no guarantee that the factors determining fertility decisions will remain constant. Moreover, as individuals gain experience with parenthood, it is reasonable to expect that their relative preferences for it and for other activities will change. Becker (1960) and others[6] have been criticized for assuming that couples at the onset of marriage make deterministic plans for the life course that include number of children, labour force participation, education decisions, and so on (Bagozzi and Van Loo, 1978a). Namboodiri (1974, 1972, 1979, 1983) has long argued that economic models of fertility should be explicitly sequential and should focus on the short-run determination of the next birth.

---

[6] For example, Willis (1973).

Even though a case[7] can be made for the utility of static models they clearly "... cannot address some of the most important empirical questions in current debates regarding future trends of birthrates, such as whether recent declines in fertility are the result of changes in the timing of births or in desired completed fertility" (Moffitt, 1984a, p. 30). Furthermore, the use of static theory to model the fertility-labour force participation nexus is compromized by the inherently dynamic and sequential nature of that behavioural relationship.

13.2.3. Measurement issues: theory versus data

The data used by economists to test their models are rarely entirely suitable to the task. Instead, the literature exhibits a widespread use of inappropriate proxies for theoretical variables with little attempt to justify either their use or relevance (Bulatao, 1986; Bagozzi and Van Loo, 1979). Moreover, even when appropriate "objective" variables such as wages, incomes, or prices are available, they may not be truly appropriate. Easterlin *et al.* (1980) among others[8] have argued that couples make decisions based on *perceived* or *expected* values rather than on actual market values.

Many potentially important variables are ignored because they are not routinely available. For example, reproductive decisions have long-range costs and benefits that must be adequately characterized and measured. Not only are these costs and benefits not usually measured, but the implicit *discount rates* that individuals apply to them are ignored even though evidence exists of systematic differences among individuals.[9] Likewise, reproductive behaviour involves significant risks and uncertainty with respect to contraception and the outcome of pregnancies; however, micro-economic analyses of fertility rarely try to incorporate analyses of risk-taking behaviour and attitudes toward uncertainty (Canlas, 1981).

Perhaps most controversial is the issue of the direct measurement of preferences. Economists have traditionally been reluctant to rely on preferences to explain behaviour because they have no theory of taste formation (Michael and Becker, 1973); moreover, economic research is often argued to "reveal" preferences through the analysis of differential behaviour without

---

[7] See, Turchi (1975, pp. 7-8).
[8] See, Bagozzi and Van Loo (1978a, 1979).
[9] See, Hausman (1979), Thaler and Shefrin (1981), and Fuchs (1986).

recourse to the direct (and unreliable) measurement of preferences. Critics point out that omission of measured preferences from empirical analyses reduces explanatory power and richness at a minimum[10] but can, if preferences vary systematically with wages and income, lead to biased estimates of taste parameters (Turchi, 1984).

Finally, because of the lack of appropriate data, the economic models are often estimated with proxies for economic variables such as education, occupation, or race that are likely to reflect taste differentials also. The reliability of interpretation of estimated parameters is, therefore, questionable.[11] Although economists have traditionally been reluctant to measure and incorporate preferences directly, the reluctance is not well grounded, and the experience of other disciplines, social psychology, political science, and sociology suggests that it is both desirable and feasible to measure preferences directly (Sen, 1973).

13.2.4. Contextual and non-economic factors

Commenting on Becker and Barro's "radically atomistic conception of society" (1986), Paul David (1986, p. 78) characterizes their view of the economy "... as a large sea surrounding many family islands ..." and society "... as the aggregation of individuals who, being stuck on these islands, remain forever isolated from the effects of actions taken by anyone other than the forebears of their lineage." David's concern for the individualistic nature of the micro-economic models of fertility is shared by many commentators. Leibenstein (1974, 1979) argues that micro-economic models of fertility often give short shrift to the non-economic motivations that affect behaviour and ignore the social constraints that limit parents' behaviour in rearing their children. Bagozzi and Van Loo (1979) complain that because theories of fertility have tended to develop in separate disciplines, they are narrow in scope and explanatory power when applied to actual behaviour. They note that fertility is a behaviour that overlaps disciplines and needs a multi-disciplinary focus.[12]

---

[10] See, Bagozzi and Van Loo (1978a), Easterlin *et al.* (1980, esp. p. 85).

[11] Even when variables such as income are available, they often do not have the expected effect on fertility. Thornton (1978) demonstrates that a simple model of the income effect will not suffice. Becker and Lewis (1973) propose one explanation for the complicated effect of income upon fertility.

[12] See also, Bulatao (1986).

Research on reproductive behaviour should concentrate on the ways in which individual decisions are influenced by the social and economic environment. Micro-economic fertility models too often focus exclusively on the impact of the economic environment to the exclusion of other external influences.[13] Although there are important differences between the sociological and economic approaches to fertility research (Namboodiri, 1978), their roles are essentially complementary (Oberschall and Leifer, 1986). Perhaps the most important feature of the micro-economic model is its untapped potential as an integrative framework for fertility analysis.[14] The following sections will present a micro-economic model that illustrates how social-demographic and social-psychological insights can be included in a resource allocation model. Moreover, the model's usefulness in linking individuals to the wider socio-economic context will be explored.

13.2.5. Simplicity versus complexity

Many students of reproductive behaviour see it as a very complex process and criticize the micro-economic models for making it too simple. For example, normative constraints on fertility and child-rearing practises are too often ignored which leads to an unrealistic picture of the choices available and behaviour exhibited.[15] Some economists avoid dealing with differential norms and preferences by "... incorporating socioeconomic variables in the technology of household production [of child quality] ... ",[16] but what is the "technology" of child-rearing but the set of norm-influenced preferences that guide parental behaviour ?

Micro-economic theory offers many advantages in the study of human fertility:

1.   it emphasizes that parenthood involves a significant reallocation of life-cycle resources;

---

[13] Their success, however, is limited even with respect to this narrower focus. Because of the data problems and inadequate specification of models mentioned previously, interpretation of empirical results as the effects of the *economic* environment is often problematic.

[14] Namboodiri (1972a, 1972b, 1978) and Turchi (1975, 1981, 1984) examine and exhibit this potential.

[15] Kiser (1979, p. 284), Leibenstein (1980), Duesenberry (1960), Canlas (1981).

[16] Keeley (1975).

2. it identifies the *immediate decision* factors such as income, wages, prices, and preferences that must directly affect the demand for children;

3. it delineates the causal paths through which these decision factors must be influenced by the social and economic environment;

4. it offers the possibility of rigorously derived testable hypotheses concerning reproductive behaviour.

Economists often focus on the mathematical derivation of hypotheses at the expense of the other benefits of the theory, and this typically involves simplification of the models to gain analytical tractability. Simplification often involves loss of correspondence with reality,[17] and the tendency to assume away the messiness of behaviour to achieve analytical tidiness may have fatal consequences when the subject is fertility. In any case, micro-economic theory has a potentially more important function as a starting point for selecting interesting variables for analysis (Larsson, 1977), and the approach described below uses it as a framework to integrate the social and psychological, as well as economic, dimensions into a more comprehensive analysis of reproductive behaviour and female labour force participation.

13.3. The demand for completed family size

Reproductive behaviour is a complex process that occurs over a significant part of a couple's life course. Achieving an equilibrium completed family size by necessity involves a series of decisions that, over an extended period, lead to the long-term result; however, for couples who actively limit their family size below the biologically attainable maximum, long-term goals likely influence short-term behaviour. The micro-economic model is potentially very useful in understanding the factors that determine long-term family size targets; moreover, it can be used to understand short-term sequential behaviours that occur at least partly in response to longer term goals.

---

[17] See, for example, Georgescu-Roegen (1970) and David (1986, p. 79).

13.3.1. Measurement of family size preferences

The concept of "demand" is central to the micro-economic analysis of fertility. Economists from Adam Smith on have emphasized the difference between *desire* for an economic commodity and the *demand* for it. The latter refers, of course, to the amount of the commodity that a person would actually purchase given its price, the prices of substitutes, and his or her income. "Demand" usually refers to a behaviour that is *observed* as opposed to an attitude that is not. Moreover, the preference functions that economists use are usually assumed to be continuous and differentiable and to have a single global maximum so that solutions in the neighbourhood of the maximum tend to be more preferred than solutions far from it.

Measurement of the quantity of children demanded at a point during a woman's reproductive life cycle is complicated by a number of features of human reproduction. First, because children generally can only be acquired sequentially over an extended period of time, the target family size that a woman chooses at any point before the end of her fecund period is in essence a "notional demand", that is, a demand incapable of being instantaneously realized.[18] The notional demand for children is itself worthy of study because (1) it is often stable over the reproductive life cycle, and (2) it may guide the short-run reproductive behaviours that lead eventually to completed family size.

Second, family size preference functions cannot necessarily be assumed to be well behaved in the sense just described. One woman who prefers three children may prefer two as a second best alternative while another who prefers three may prefer four as a second best alternative. In terms of the demand for completed family size, the two women are the same; however, in terms of the *fertility control behaviour* they exhibit during the reproductive life cycle, they may differ considerably. Another woman may prefer no children, but two children if she has any. If she experiences a contraceptive failure she may then opt for two children, not one child. It is, therefore, important to

---

[18] The concept of "notional demand" is borrowed from disequilibrium theory in macro-economics, where it implies a quantity that would be demanded at a given price in a certain market if there were not some constraint to market clearing in that or related markets. "Notional demand" as used here implies that a woman may demand a certain number of children at a point in her reproductive life cycle but for biological reasons she is unable to achieve it instantaneously.

understand the structure of preferences for family size in order better to understand short-range demand behaviour and the contraceptive behaviour practised by women.[19]

13.3.2. A notional demand model

Picture a married woman at some age (a) in her reproductive life cycle. Because children arrive sequentially in a biologically delimited period of years, a woman who seeks actively to choose her completed family size needs to engage in some planning well before the onset of subfecundity. Planning is necessary to avoid exceeding the target family size or to allow sufficient time to achieve it.

What factors determine a woman's target or notional demand for children ? The micro-economic model reflects the economist's view that, because children require large amounts of economic resources, the choice of family size must be treated as a resource allocation decision. Because children in industrial countries are generally not expected to provide economic support to their parents, the family size decision is broadly analogous to other consumption decisions, and the same set of factors should determine the outcome of those decisions.[20] These factors are the decision maker's relative preferences for parenthood versus alternative consumption and work activities, the prices of those activities and the level of resources available to consume over the life cycle.

The objective function

Formally, the wife is represented as maximizing a utility function which represents the preference weightings she gives to alternative activities at that particular point in her reproductive life cycle:

$$U_a = U_a(K, N; PR^s_{k:n}).$$

---

[19] See, McClelland (1983) for a review of the issues surrounding demand for children measures. See also Coombs (1974) and Terhune and Kaufman (1973).

[20] The analogy between fertility and consumption is not perfect: (1) children arrive sequentially over an extended period of time and the demand for them cannot instantaneously be realized; (2) children may be "purchased" as the unintended outcome of another activity; (3) fertility decisions, unlike most consumer durable purchases, cannot be reversed.

U_a is the woman's perceived utility level at age a, K is the total number of children she might choose over the reproductive life cycle, N is an indicator of the level of all non-child-rearing-related activities, and $PR_{k:n}^s$ is an indicator of her relative preferences for child-rearing versus all other activities.[21]

The decision maker's problem is to find the pair $\{K^*, N^*\}$, K = 0, ..., MAX, that will maximize the utility function and then to undertake behaviour that will lead to the optimal family size, K^*. N does not represent an alternate commodity as much as it does a share of life-cycle resources. Couples must make their final long-range fertility decisions long before much of the cost of child-rearing is actually paid and alternative activities are undertaken. Consequently, early determinations of the notional demand for children really involve dividing life-cycle family resources into a child-rearing and a non-child-rearing component. The mix of commodities in the second component does not have to be known or specified in order to make that division; indeed, it cannot since fertility decisions must be finalized relatively early in the life cycle.[22]

The preference indicator is normally not included in the utility function since the functional operator stands for it; however, it is included here specifically to emphasize (1) that relative preferences may systematically change over the reproductive life cycle, and (2) that they may differ systematically among women of varying socioeconomic characteristics.

Economists often ignore these two features of preferences and assume that constant and uniform[23] preference structures will be revealed by actual

---

[21] "All other activities" includes preferences for work and career at this stage. Distinction between work and other non-market activities is not necessary at this level of analysis. Section 4 illustrates the short-run situation in which a woman actually has to choose between work, child-rearing, and other non-market activities.

[22] The budgeting problem here is similar to a two-stage budgeting procedure in which households first allocate income optimally between two commodity groups based upon aggregate price indices and then optimally allocate each budget allotment among commodities in that specific group (Blackorby *et al.*, 1970; Blackorby *et al.*, 1978, ch. 5; Gorman, 1959; Strotz, 1957, 1959); however, in the present case many of the same market commodities are contained in each group, and it is not clear that the same necessary and sufficient conditions for price aggregation obtain.

[23] For econometric purposes, all that is required is that variations in the preference structure are randomly and independently distributed with respect to the specified determinants of demand.

behaviour even if they are not measured directly. Empirical work performed under this assumption will, if it is incorrect, lead to biased inferences about the factors that determine completed family size. Moreover, although psychological factors in the form of relative preferences clearly play a central role in resource allocation decision making, their importance is often understated because economists deal with them only indirectly through the restrictive assumptions just mentioned. Integrative and multi-disciplinary research should relax the constancy and uniformity of preference assumptions in order to understand more fully the complex relationship among preferences, prices, wages, and social status.

The long-range budget constraint

The budget share devoted to child-rearing is constrained by the life-time economic resources available to the couple. The life-cycle resource constraint is:

$$P_k^s K + P_n N = I = V + W_w \cdot T_w + W_h \cdot T_h,$$

where P_k^s is a scalar representing the discounted present value of expected expenditures on market goods and parental time made on one child over the child's life in the family:

$$P_k^s = \int_0^{\tau(s)} p^s(\alpha) \cdot e^{-\rho(s)\alpha} \, d\alpha.$$

Its value depends upon the value of annual expenditures, $p^s(\alpha)$; the length of time, α ranging from 0 to $\tau(s)$, that the parents support the child; the discount rate, $\rho(s)$, at which the decision maker discounts future expenditures; and the time shape of the stream of expenditures.[24] The indicator, s, marks those components of the price of a child that might be expected to vary systematically with the social status of the parents. It provides a link with society's restrictions on parental behaviour that sociologists commonly call norms, and its significance to the theory will be described below.

---

[24] In the United States actual parental money expenditures on children are concentrated in the ages twelve and over (Turchi, 1983, ch. 4), and parental time contributions are concentrated at the early ages (Turchi, 1986, ch. 5).

The quantity, P_nN, represents the share of potential income that is tentatively allocated to non-child-rearing activities. The decision maker acts as if she is making a preliminary division of potential income between child-rearing and all other activities. Once children start arriving in the family, the composition of the child-rearing share becomes more defined; however, the composition of alternative expenditures can be expected to remain relatively fluid, with great possibilities for substitution among activities so early in the life cycle. Consequently, P_n can be expected to play a much less prominent role in determining the notional demand for children than P_k^S, the price of a child.

The right-hand side of the budget constraint describes the potential income, I, of the family. It is the woman's expectation of the maximum discounted value of economic resources available over the life cycle. V is the present value of expected life-time family wealth from previous work and from previous and expected future non-labour sources. T_w and T_h represent vectors of time available to the wife and husband, respectively, over the life cycle, and W_w and W_h are corresponding discounted expected wage vectors.

The budget constraint emphasizes the necessity of parents' making fertility decisions (1) well before desired family size is achieved, and (2) well before the bulk of the costs of child-rearing are incurred. Thus, the decision maker must look into the future and weigh the future costs and benefits of parenthood. Often the discount rate, $\rho(s)$, is assumed to be uniform across individuals; however, evidence[25] suggests that it varies systematically. If it does, parents facing identical streams of future income and expenditures will perceive them to be different, and their family size decisions and reproductive behaviour may also diverge systematically.

The demand function

A formal characterization of the woman's choice of target family size involves the maximization of the utility function subject to the life-time budget constraint.[26] The decision problem is to

---

[25] See, Hausman (1979), Thaler and Shefrin (1981), and Fuchs (1986).

[26] As is common, the discrete nature of the choice is ignored here for expositional purposes; however, the econometrics of demand function estimation require that the discreteness of family size options be considered.

Maximize: $U_a = U_a(K, N; PR_{k:n})$

Subject to: $P_k^S K + P_n N = I = V + W_w \cdot T_w + W_h \cdot T_h$.

Forming the Lagrangean function and differentiating leads to the first-order conditions:[27]

$$\partial U_a / \partial K - \lambda P_k^S = 0$$

$$\partial U_a / \partial N - \lambda P^n = 0$$

$$- P_k^S - P_n N + I = 0.$$

With an explicit functional form for the utility function, it is possible to solve for the optimum number of children in terms of the price of a child, a price index for alternative activities, and potential income. In its absence we have the general form of the demand function:

$$K^D = f(P_k^S, P_n, I; PR_{k:n}^S).$$

The demand for children, K^D, is a function of four "proximate decision factors": (1) P_k^S, the perceived price of a child; (2) P_n, the price index of alternative activities; (3) I, potential income; and (4) $PR_{k:n}^S$, relative preferences for child-rearing versus a composite alternative. Each of these proximate decision factors relates directly to the choice problem of a single and specific decision maker. They are all psychological variables, being expectations or perceptions, but three of the four are actually perceptions of economic variables. Economic models often substitute actual market prices for perceived prices, but this appears to be especially problematic with respect to the notional demand for children.

Under this economic model the proximate decision factors represent the only paths through which variables external to the decision maker can affect her free choice of target family size. Figure 1 shows how the micro-economic model forces all external influences to operate through the budget constraint

---

[27] Ignore for the moment the possible dependence of the perceived price of a child upon the number of children chosen.

via prices and potential income or through relative preferences. Almost invariably analyses of the demand for children, lacking measures of these appropriate theoretical variables, resort to proxies such as race, education, religion, occupation, etc., to explain the decisions. However, use of these proxies can lead to conflicting interpretations of empirical results. A negative coefficient on "education", for example, may signify "wage effects" to an economist or "taste effects" to a sociologist, when it is in fact indirectly influencing both wages and tastes.[28]

The basic demand model of figure 1 provides the framework through which the analysis can be expanded to incorporate a variety of influences from the commodity and labour markets and from the normative environment within which the decision maker resides. After the origin of P_k^s is explored further, the demand model will be expanded to serve as a more comprehensive vehicle for the analysis of fertility decisions.

Figure 1. Basic notional demand model illustrating the effect of
"proximate decision factors"

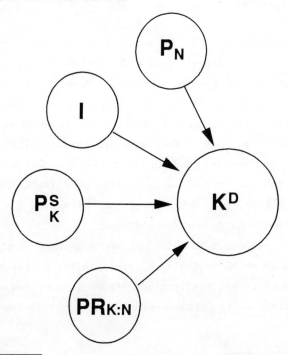

---

[28] Cochrane (1979) provides a comprehensive survey of the complexities of the education-fertility link.

13.3.3. Production technology and the price of a child

The notional demand model specifies that the demand for children is determined in part by the perceived or expected price of a child. This formulation reflects the view that parental child-rearing inputs are significantly determined by social norms and standards which vary systematically across the status hierarchy. Since social status is related to education and occupation, which also are important determinants of potential income it is likely that the perceived price of a child is systematically related to potential income.

The notional demand model differs from the more common "quantity-quality" model[29] in that it views the price of a child as a determinant of the demand for children, while the latter approach assumes that the quantity and "quality" of children are chosen simultaneously.[30] This assumption, along with the assumption of uniform preferences and child-quality production technology across households, means that the demand for children can be estimated without any direct reference to the resources required for child-rearing.

The view embodied here is that parents base their demand for children on a previously determined price of a child which is systematically related both to the economic environment (labour and commodity markets) and to the social normative environment. This approach must, consequently, pay much more attention to the measurement and specification of child-rearing behaviour, but it also offers a richer set of paths connecting individuals to the economic and social environments. Since a primary purpose of the study of reproductive decision making is, or should be, the analysis of how individuals respond to the environment in which they live, the approach proposed here offers attractive possibilities for extending our knowledge along these lines.

The household technology of child production

Let us characterize the "technology" by which a woman expects to raise her children as a perceived "production function" that relates the quantities of market goods and services and parental time required to raise children:

---

[29] See, for example, Becker (1960), Willis (1973), and Schultz (1976).

[30] Assume "quality" is an indicator of expenditure per child and therefore is analogous to the "price" of a child. The literature is not clear about just what the quality of a child is.

$\phi^s(K,x,t) = 0.$

K is the number of children, x is a vector of market goods and services (e.g., food, clothing, housing, education, etc.) over the entire period of child-rearing, and t is a vector of parental time inputs over the child-rearing period. The production function determines the quantities of each input used to produce a given number of children and it also specifies a decision maker's perceptions regarding the degree of substitutability among inputs in the child-rearing process.

Where does this production function (or the production function for child quality) come from ? For families at minimum levels of subsistence the required inputs are *biologically determined*; however, for most children living in the industrial world, the technology is *socially determined*. The production function sets minimum acceptable standards for child-rearing and these standards are likely to be a function of social status.[31] The theoretical approach proposed here offers a linkage among the social and economic environment and important proximate determinants of fertility.

The perceived price of a child

Given the minimum standards implicit in the production function, assume that a decision maker will produce children in a least costly manner:

Minimize: $C = p \cdot x + w \cdot t$

Subject to: $\phi^s(\underline{K},x,t) = 0,$

where, p is a vector of discounted expected market prices, w is a vector of expected wages[32] and $\underline{K}$ indicates that the minimization is for a particular family size.

Minimization of costs implies a cost function that depends on family size, prices, and wages,

---

[31] See, Becker (1981, p. 107) for an implicit recognition that even in the quantity-quality model there is some floor on the expenditures that parents make on their children.

[32] Actually, these are expected *shadow* wages since the time used in child-rearing is non-market time.

$$C = C^s(K,p,w),$$

and the perceived price of a child would be

$$P_k^s = C/K = F^s(K,p,w) \qquad \text{or} \qquad = F^s(p,w),$$

if the decision maker believes there are economies of scale in child-rearing.[33]

The perceived price of a child is, therefore, a function of expected market prices, shadow wages which are in turn related to market wages, and the normative standards that parents bring to child-rearing. The perceived price of a child may or may not be a function of target family size. Turchi (1983, 1986) has shown that *actual* child-rearing expenses per child are a function of family size;[34] however, individual expectations may diverge from actuality.

13.3.4. Notional demand in an economic, social, and psychological context

The micro-economic demand model might to many seem to be excessively individualistic, since external forces - markets, social norms, peer group preferences, laws and regulations, etc. - appear to play no role in the selection of the woman's target family size; however, nothing could be further from the case. This model actually is capable of specifying an exhaustive set of paths through which contextual factors influence individual-level decisions. Figure 2 illustrates the linkages between an individual's decision problem and her economic, social, political, and natural environment.

Space allows only a brief survey of the paths through which an individual's decisions are influenced by the various communities within which she resides; however, it will be clear from this survey that the potential environmental constraints affecting an individual's "free" fertility decision can be multi-faceted indeed.

---

[33] A national survey conducted by me asked respondents to report whether they believe that child-rearing is a constant, increasing, or decreasing returns to scale activity: 25.6 per cent believed costs per child would remain constant with increasing family size, 31.5 per cent thought costs would fall to some degree, and 42.9 per cent thought costs would rise.

[34] See also, Lazear and Michael (1988).

Figure 2. Contextual model of a woman's notional demand for children

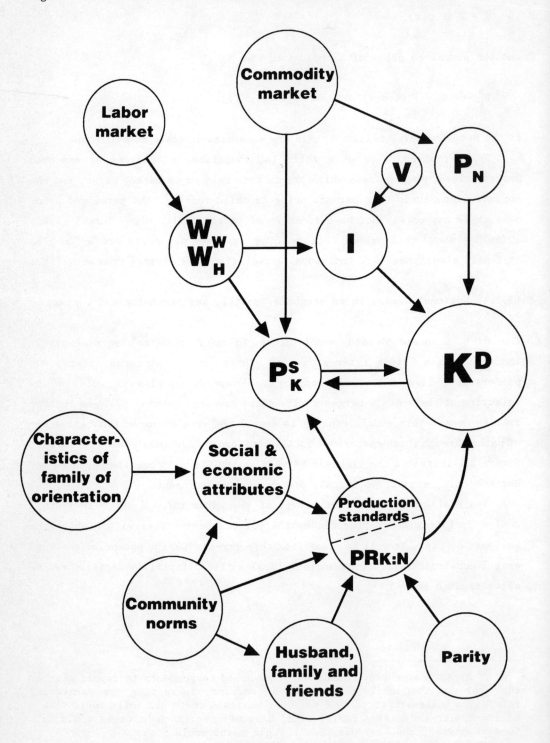

I have already argued that a woman's relative preferences for children can be systematically related to her social attributes and through them to the larger social context. This assertion certainly does not trouble most non-economists, but the vast majority of micro-level decision theoretic research in economics ignores this possibility by assuming preferences in a population to be uniform and fixed,[35] thereby foreclosing *a priori* a major source of influence from society and culture operating through decision makers' preferences.

Figure 2 suggests that a woman's preferences for children versus other activities, $PR_{k:n}$, may be systematically linked to her own social attributes, as well as to the normative pressure exerted by husband, family, friends, and the social community of which she is a member. Moreover, another part of her preference structure which plays an important role in fertility decisions is the set of preferences she brings to the child-rearing role ("Production Standards"). These preferences can also be normatively influenced in the same manner as her preferences for children versus other activities.

Models that ignore the systematic variation in the demand for children which stems from membership in different groups suffer, at a minimum, loss of explanatory power. More importantly, however, they run the risk of simply being wrong because of the misspecification bias that is inherent in their incompletely specified view of the determinants of demand. In figure 2, social factors affect not only preferences but also such economic variables as the price of a child, P_k^S, and household potential income, I, operating through wage rates. Omission of direct measures of preferences and child-rearing standards leads directly to bias in the coefficients of those variables that *are* included in the model.

Many students of fertility have used social attributes such as race, education, occupation, or religious affiliation as explanatory variables in their empirical models. These attributes do not directly determine reproductive decisions, but they influence variables that do. Unfortunately, without a well-specified decision theory, interpretation of such analyses is problematic. For economists these social attributes are proxies for (missing) wages or prices, but for sociologists they may represent normative influences on behaviour operating through preferences.

---

[35] Or, perhaps, randomly and independently distributed with respect to the other proximate decision factors.

The micro-economic model makes clear the sorts of variables that directly affect allocative decisions such as fertility, and it (or another explicitly decision theoretic model) is essential for a proper understanding of the determinants and outcomes of decision processes. In addition, the micro-economic model offers the (generally unexploited) advantage of pinpointing the sources of external influence for individual decisions. After all, social scientists are generally interested in how the wider society and economy affect the individual, and an individual-level theory is a prerequisite for constructing the network of relationships that determines a person's place in the economic and social system.

Finally, figure 2 makes it clear that an individual is not affected simply by a single "community." Rather, her decisions are affected simultaneously by a number of different communities. On the economic side, both the labour and commodity markets, which do not need to be coterminous, have separate effects on the decision process. The social pressures that shape preferences and child-rearing standards also emanate from the various social, religious, or racial communities of which she is a member. Consequently, the demand for children is considered to be the result of a complex interaction of forces emerging from a number of different contexts, both social and economic, that probably cannot be studied effectively in isolation.

13.4. Fertility and labour force participation

The biologically mandated sequentiality of fertility prohibits instantaneous achievement of target family size and complicates the fertility-labour force participation relationship. A woman makes labour force participation decisions continually throughout her reproductive age span, and her long-range fertility goals are contingent upon them as are the more immediate economic and social conditions that change continually. Students of the fertility-labour force participation relationship have approached it from a number of different perspectives: (1) current (or cumulative) labour force participation versus current family size,[36] (2) life-cycle fertility versus life-cycle labour force

---

[36] See, for example, Smith-Lovin and Tickamyer (1978), Cain and Dooley (1976), and Dooley (1982).

participation,[37] (3) optimal control models of fertility and labour force participation,[38] and (4) multi-period sequential models.[39]

Of course the appropriate time frame for analysis depends somewhat upon the specific objectives of the particular research; however, three different aspects of time are potentially relevant:

1. *Age of Woman*. There is a "typical" age profile of a married woman's labour force participation and fertility that is arguably stable across cohorts. This age profile is determined significantly by the biological course of fecundity between ages fifteen to forty-four, but it can be modified by trends in preferences for the timing of births and labour force participation.

2. *Cohort Effects*. Preferences might vary systematically by cohort so as to distort the age profile of reproduction and work. Use of data from many cohorts, as is often done in cross-sectional statistical analyses, may lead to biases in estimation if care is not taken to account for these cohort effects. An example of cohort effects might be the apparent trend toward later childbearing and earlier establishment of careers among American women in post-1960 cohorts.

3. *Period Effects*. The forces that determine *actual behaviour* in a given period are often exogenous to the decision maker and serve to distort the (preference modified) "typical" age profile of fertility and labour force participation. For example, recessions that lead to a husband's unemployment may force a wife to stay at work although both she and her husband desire for her to quit work and begin a family. Namboodiri (1972a) has long argued forcefully that the "life cycle" is actually a series of short-run episodes that must be modelled as such.

The model presented in figure 3 reflects my choice to emphasize the interplay of period effects and the long-range or notional demand for children in producing a woman's short-run supply of hours to the labour market and the intensity of demand for a pregnancy in the current time period. The model

---

[37] Waite and Stolzenberg (1973), Stolzenberg and Waite (1977), Willis (1973), Carliner *et al.* (1984), Fleisher and Rhodes (1979), Rosenzweig and Wolpin (1980).

[38] Moffitt (1984a).

[39] Namboodiri (1972a), Rosenzweig and Schultz (1985), and Hotz and Miller (1988).

reflects my conviction that the fertility-labour force participation relationship must be treated as a short-run behaviour contingent upon long-range
plans.[40] Again, this model's purpose is to emphasize the opportunities for an
interdisciplinary approach to a comprehensive explanation of the fertility-
work interaction.

The model contains two dependent variables: the wife's supply of hours
during time period t, and the intensity of her demand for a pregnancy during
the same period.[41] These two endogenous variables[42] are specified as being
jointly determined by a nexus of *current* social and economic variables, and
in the case of pregnancy intentions by the notional (or long-range) demand
for children. In this sense both labour force participation and short-run
fertility intentions are mutually determined but do not mutually determine
each other.[43]

The woman's supply of hours to the labour market has three direct determinants: current exogenous income, the woman's current wage rate, and the
current shadow value of her time. Exogenous current income includes income
from non-human assets (financial and real) as well as the husband's labour
income.[44] It depends fundamentally upon current economic conditions in the
labour market (unemployment rate), the financial market (stock and bond
prices), the housing market (real estate income), etc. The woman's current
wage rate also depends upon current labour market conditions and it depends
also upon the social and economic attributes that determine her productivity
at work.

The shadow value of a wife's time is a latent psychological measure of
the value she places on her time at home. Its value depends upon her *current*
preferences for work versus pregnancy, which may be quite different from her
life-cycle preferences, the current number, age, and sex of children in the
family, and on the availability and quality of child care from outside the

---

[40] See Hill and Stafford (1985a) for empirical support for the notion that
long-range fertility plans affect the short-run relationship between fertility
and labour force behaviour.

[41] The latter variable might be measured as a dichotomous one in the data
(e.g, "Are you intending to become pregnant this year ?") requiring use of a
probit equation in a systems context.

[42] A third supply of hours to non-market, non-parental activities could
have been added but is omitted here for simplicity.

[43] Support for this view of the relationship comes in papers by Bagozzi
and Van Loo (1982, 1988), Van Loo and Bagozzi (1984), and Moffitt (1984).

[44] In the United States numerous studies have demonstrated that husband's
labour income is independent of wife's work effort.

home.[45] Figure 3 shows how normative pressure emanating from the husband, family and friends, and other sources can differentially affect women in varying social milieus.

The wife's demand for a pregnancy depends directly upon her current preferences for work versus parenthood which depend in turn upon the biological factors that influence reproduction (age, fecundity), the number, age, and sex of her children, and the normative pressure for work or pregnancy that she receives from husband, family, and friends. In addition, of course, the notional demand for children influences her current demand for a pregnancy which implies that this current behaviour is also influenced by that complex network of influences pictured in figure 2.

Figure 3. Wife's supply of labour market hours and demand for a
          pregnancy in year t

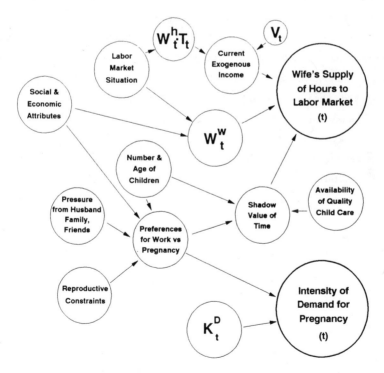

---

[45] Many empirical studies of female labour force participation ignore this variable completely or use incomplete measures such as "number of children under age five" as proxies.

13.5. Conclusions

This essay has argued that utility maximization theory can serve a potentially valuable role as an integrating framework for the interdisciplinary study of fertility and labour force participation behaviour. In the industrial world, both fertility and work are generally undertaken as the consequence of deliberate decisions; each involves the expenditure of economic resources and leads to psychic and/or economic returns. The micro-economic model as normally used focusses on decision makers' responses to the economic environment - labour and commodity markets - but it also offers the opportunity to integrate social, psychological and normative variables to produce a comprehensive model. Figures 2 and 3 offer suggestions for how this integration might take place.

   Although not discussed here, it should be clear that a comprehensive model of fertility and labour force participation makes significantly greater data demands than analyses with a narrower disciplinary focus. The integrative model pays much more attention to *measurement* of commonly unmeasured theoretical variables. Economists tend to stand back from the measurement of preferences, a reticence that sociologists and psychologists find unwarranted. On the other hand, the model also suggests that behavioural models that fail to measure and include in analysis the economic constraints that accompany allocative behaviours such as fertility and labour force participation are, in their own ways, equally open to bias arising from specification error. The data collection tasks implied by the integrative models of this essay are not insignificant, but they offer the possibility of a significantly richer understanding of two of society's most fundamental socioeconomic processes.

Part V
Towards a Better Understanding of the Relationship between Female Labour Market Behaviour and Fertility

TOWARDS A BETTER UNDERSTANDING OF THE RELATIONSHIP BETWEEN FEMALE LABOUR MARKET BEHAVIOUR AND FERTILITY[46]

Jacques J. Siegers
Economisch Instituut / CIAV
Rijksuniversiteit Utrecht
Domplein 24
3512 JE UTRECHT
The Netherlands

14.1. Introduction

How can we gain more insight into the relationship between female labour market behaviour and fertility ? One matter is clear: a purely monodisciplinary approach will not do. In organizing the workshop on "Female Labour Market Behaviour and Fertility" this point of view solved at least one problem: we did not have to make a choice between disciplines; we took them all. As the reader will have noticed, this is only partially true. Given the lack of time and money we left out, for example, the entire field of biology. We were well aware that the implication was that the workshop would focus mainly on the demand for children and much less so or hardly at all on the supply side.

However, the choice for an interdisciplinary approach did not only solve a problem, it also raised one: how is it possible to integrate demography, econometrics, economics, psychology, and sociology within one workshop ? For this, we needed a theoretical framework. As has been mentioned before in the present volume, the framework we chose was the rational-choice framework. For an economist this is a natural choice, because economic analysis, and especially microeconomic analysis, is in fact a specification of the rational-choice framework. The central thesis of the workshop, as well as my present paper, is that the general rational-choice framework offers an ideal opportunity to combine the advantages of both economics and the other social sciences, namely to enrich the rather bare but formal and elegant economic models with psychological and sociological insights. Moreover, biological aspects can easily be incorporated in this framework. Before I go into detail

---

[46] This paper draws partly on my PhD-thesis *Arbeidsaanbod en kindertal: een micro-economische analyse* ("Labour supply and fertility: a microeconomic approach"), Groningen, 1985, and partly on my paper "Towards the construction of interdisciplinary theoretical models to explain demographic behaviour", in: C.A. Hazeu and G.A.B. Frinking (eds.), *Emerging issues in demographic research*, Amsterdam: Elsevier, 1990.

about this thesis, I will present concise evaluations of the economic approaches to labour supply and fertility, respectively.

14.2. An evaluation of the economic approach to labour supply

In the period before the rise of neoclassical theory, treatises on individual labour supply were rather impressionistic in nature. The answers to the then much discussed question whether the labour supply curve is forward bending (i.e. a higher wage rate induces a larger supply of labour) or backward bending (i.e. a higher wage rate induces a smaller supply of labour) seems to have rested on the vision the authors had on society, rather than on empirical research (Sandy, 1977). The rudimentary empirical analyses of Adam Smith (1776/1970, Part I, pp. 72-75) prove to be exceptions.

The start and development of the neoclassical theory of labour supply produced a theoretical framework for a systematic analysis of several aspects of labour supply. The first marginalistic foundations of this framework were already visible at the end of the 19th century: an adequate apparatus of concepts and, first partly implicit, the hard core and the protective belt of the neoclassical research programme, as these elements of scientific research programmes have been coined by Lakatos (1970; see also Latsis, 1976). An important milestone was reached when Robbins (1930) demonstrated that it cannot be deduced from economic theory alone whether the labour supply curve is forward or backward bending.

The change from cardinal to ordinal utility analysis in neoclassical theory provided new impulses to the development of the theoretical framework. A series of theorems were deduced which lend themselves for empirical testing. Furthermore, several theoretical advances were reached, including those reached by acknowledging that individual labour supply generally takes place within the context of a household. This led to analyses of the interdependency of labour supply of partners within a household, as well as to an extension of the labour-leisure choice to a choice between labour, leisure and housework. But, above all, ordinal utility analysis proved to be a very useful instrument for the analysis of a broad range of policy questions, like those with respect to the effects on labour supply of taxes, social insurance, entry costs, and institutional restrictions regaring the length of the working-week. The importance of this instrument becomes immediately clear if one tries to conceive how to study such policy questions in the absence of the neoclassical analytical framework.

From the very beginning, the neoclassical theory of labour supply was part of the neoclassical research programme. This embedment of the theory of labour supply in the neoclassical research programme has had a number of important consequences. In the first place it enabled one to study labour supply as part of a system of interdependencies. This in turn made it possible to study a variety of phenomena, e.g. labour supply and fertility, within a single theoretical framework. The second consequence has been that the development of the theory of labour supply was strongly influenced and furthered by developments within the neoclassical research programme. Examples are the derivation of the Slutsky equations and accompanying theorems, and the inclusion of labour supply in both the systems analysis and the life-cycle analysis of consumer demand. A third consequence has been that empirical research into labour supply was given greater impetus, due to the fact that the neoclassical theory has generally proved to be a stimulus to empirical research.

Developments within the neoclassical theory of labour supply appears to be characterized by a desire to increase the theory's own plausibility (Siegers, 1985, pp. 92-94). To some extent, this desire can be interpreted as an attempt to incorporate into the present mathematically oriented labour supply models, aspects of labour supply that have been lost from sight since the days of Marshall.

14.3. An evaluation of the economic approach to fertility

The economic theory of fertility is rooted in the work of Malthus. Although it does not follow naturally from his analyses (in contrast to what e.g. Andorka, 1978, pp. 15-17, purports), researchers have concluded that Malthus considered per capita income to be positively related to the number of births. However, empirical research has generally failed to demonstrate such a relationship; more often than not, even a negative relationship has been found (Van de Kaa and Moors, 1982). This has inspired many authors to construct models that both fit the neoclassical research programme and are compatible with the obtained empirical findings. In doing so, they have assumed that the underlying relationship between fertility and income will be positive if conditions which are linked to income are kept constant. Presumably, the positive effect of income on fertility does not emerge because if income changes, other phenomena also change. According to Becker and his followers, it is because child quality rises with income that the income elasticity of fertility tends to be very small or even negative.

Most of the economic theory of fertility forms part of the New Home Economics. However, the advantages which the New Home Economics has brought for the economic theory of fertility are still small compared with, for example, the benefits which the economic theory of labour supply has derived from its incorporation into the theory of consumer behaviour (Siegers, 1985). Developments within economics in the field of the New Home Economics have been relatively limited, though I must of course point out that the New Home Economics was developed much more recently than was the theory of consumer behaviour. Moreover, empirical testing poses problems owing to the fact that, among others, when applying the New Home Economics to an explanation of fertility, phenomena are introduced into the model that are not as easily translated into variables suitable for empirical analysis as they are in the in the field that is traditionally covered by economics. An example is the problem of adequately operationalizing the previously mentioned concept of "child quality"; in a recent evaluation, Willis (1987, p. 75) speaks of an "unresolved issue" in this regard.

The economic theory of fertility has been subject to much more severe criticism than has the related economic theory of individual labour supply. A possible reason is that in the former, more stringent assumptions must be made when deriving empirically verifiable hypotheses from theory (Siegers, 1985, pp. 196-196; Siegers, 1987, p. 114). Another reason is that the role of social values and norms is deemed much more important in decision-making, by individuals and households, with regard to fertility than in decisions regarding labour supply. According to some, the options are so limited in the case of fertility that economic science has hardly any role to play; this field should be left to social demographers, so it is argued (Kinsella, 1975). This point of view is in agreement with Duesenberry's statement (1960, p. 233) that "Economics is all about how people make choices. Sociology is all about why they don't have any choices to make." Closely linked to the second is a third reason, namely that a sociology of individual labour supply hardly exists (cf. Veenman, 1983, pp. 208-209), whereas social demography has a long tradition. Thus, criticism of the economic theory of fertility is partly voiced by social demographers, who saw "their" field invaded by economists (Blake, 1967, 1968; see also Namboodiri, 1972, 1975, and Ryder, 1974).

Most of the criticism of the economic theory of fertility is directed at the assumptions it makes. However, for participants in the neoclassical research programme in the field of fertility, these assumptions belong to, in the terminology of Lakatos (1970), the hard core or the protective belt of this programme (Siegers, 1985, pp. 6 and 196). For this reason, the criticism barely seems to have influenced the development of the economic theory of fertility.

The economic theory of fertility appears to focus predominantly on determining the extent to which the research programme is capable of explaining known phenomena, including the previously mentioned negative relationship between fertility and income (Blaug, 1980, p. 248; Perlman, 1975, p. 554; Namboodiri, 1975, pp. 564 and 568). Despite this verificationist tendency, the economic theory of fertility is able to throw new light on a number of demographic phenomena. In particular, I would like to mention the consequences of Willis' interaction model for the empirical analysis and interpretation of the relationship between fertility on the one hand and the level of education of men and women on the other hand; I would also like to refer to what the theory has to say about the interpretation of what Schultz (1981, p. 230) has called "The classical problem that brings labour and population economics together", that is to say, the relationship between fertility and labour supply.

The application of the New Home Economics to the explanation of fertility yields a theoretical analytical framework from which models can be derived - with the aid of supplementary assumptions - in order to answer specific research questions (see Siegers, 1985, p. 198 and the references therein). Nevertheless, very few models that can actually be used in policy-making have as yet been developed. This is particularly true for the Netherlands, where the economic analysis of fertility is still in its infancy. In fact, this is the case for economic explanations of demographic behaviour in general, as can be illustrated by the fact that of the nine papers in the field of demographic changes and economic developments that were submitted to the Royal Netherlands Economic Association in 1987 on the occasion of its 125th anniversary, seven dealt with the economic consequences of demographic phenomena and only two attempted to provide an explanation for these phenomena (Kapteyn, 1987).

Economic theory in the field of fertility has, until now, paid relatively little attention to the decision-making process of (potential) parents. Nevertheless, this process is a crucial factor in explaining both the present and the ultimate number of children. During one's life cycle, the restrictions one faces change constantly. These restrictions can be both exogenous (e.g., involuntary unemployment) and predetermined endogenous (e.g., the current fixed costs of a household depend for a part on whether one bought a house in the past; another example: the current earning capacity depends for a part on investments made in the past in human capital, including experiences gained during employment, and so it depends on past labour force participation and on the interruption of one's career to raise children. Cf. Groot *et al.*, 1988 and forthcoming). Strictly speaking, almost every current restriction comprises a predetermined element (the probability of involuntary unemployment is determined in part by the job one has chosen in the past, which in turn may have been determined by the desired number of children, and the probability of involuntary childlessness is partly determined by delayed pregnancies in the past). With given preferences, behaviour will change as restrictions change during the course of one's life. However, restrictions and behaviour are not the only aspects that change during a lifetime: the preferences themselves change too. Both the preferences with respect to the timing of births and those with respect to the ultimate number of children change over time. Even if the desired timing and the desired number of children do not change, the preferences will at least become more defined during one's life cycle (see, e.g., Veevers' study on voluntary childlessness, 1973), until preferences and reality coincide, or else until those involved are forced to reconcile themselves to the facts (see also the theory of mental incongruity, Tazelaar, 1980).

14.4. The rational-choice framework as a basis for interdisciplinary analyses

On the basis of the evaluations of the economic approach to labour supply and fertility, three related research priorities can be formulated (Siegers, 1990):

a.   extending the economic analysis by introducing relevant factors that do not belong to the traditional field of economics (Cramer, 1986, p. 50, presents as his main conclusion with respect to priorities in economic

research: "Extending the analysis with non-economic factors has priority
over a further refinement of the theoretical specification.");

b. research into the question how the system of preferences, restrictions
and behaviour changes during the life cycle, and into the question which
determinants are responsible for these changes;

c. construction of theoretical models that can be translated into empirical
estimation models to be used in policy.

I will now elaborate the manner in which the first priority can be treated with
the help of the rational-choice framework.

In applying the "preferences - restrictions - behaviour" scheme of the
rational-choice framework to a specific research question, it is possible to
include both the specific preferences and the specific restrictions that are
generally analysed within economics, as well as the specific preferences and
the specific restrictions that tend to be examined within the other social
sciences (see also Turchi, this volume). As a consequence, data collection can
be directed towards obtaining information that enables more relationships to
be identified within one model than was possible until now, thus allowing more
behavioural aspects to be endogenized in the theoretical model and the corresponding empirical estimation models. However, this does not detract from the
principle that we should strive for parsimonious models, since the essence of
modelling is that it helps us to see the wood through the trees. And parsimony
in particular appears to be a necessary element in a research strategy that
is aimed at explaining more than one behavioural aspect.

The first step in the application of the rational-choice framework, with
a view to explaining female labour supply and fertility, is the construction
of the preference functions for both partners. Two possible general, final
preferences are physical well-being and social approval (Lindenberg, this
volume). Income or economic independence, leisure, and having children
(Niphuis-Nell, 1981; Den Bandt, 1982; Rozendal *et al.*, 1985) can be seen to
be lower level preferences, i.e. preferences that serve as instruments in
realizing the general preferences mentioned above; we can thus speak of a
hierarchy of preferences (Bagozzi, 1984). This build-up of final and intermediary preferences is entirely analogous to the relationship between
commodities on the one hand and the factors of production, time and market
goods, on the other hand in the New Home Economics. Similarly, the functional
relationships between final and intermediary preferences can, by analogy with

the New Home Economics, be called production functions. However, in this case
the functions are not technical production functions describing the technical
production process through which time and market goods are transformed into
commodities, but they are social production functions describing, for example,
how social approval, that is to say status, behavioural confirmation and
positive affect, can be obtained from, among other things, adherence to norms,
occupation and income (Lindenberg, this volume).

If we translate the "preferences - restrictions - behaviour" scheme into
a specific model, and if we know two of the three parts of the scheme and thus
of the model, then we can derive the third part. So if we know everything about
the preferences and everything about the restrictions, we can derive the
resulting behaviour. In empirical analyses, at least in much economic and
sociological research, we observe behaviour and restrictions, and preferences
are only there by implication. This raises the question whether we can try and
"observe" preferences and incorporate these preferences into our economic and
sociological models. Of course, if we do so, we "observe" all three parts of
the "preferences - restrictions - behaviour" scheme and risk introducing
inconsistencies. But should we not search for such risks, and can we not learn
from possible inconsistencies, for the purpose of improving our models ? One
can raise the objection that the measurement of preferences is not an easy task
(see, e.g., Burch, this volume; Deven and Bauwens, this volume; Spieß *et al.*,
this volume). However, this is also true for the measurement of restrictions
(such as income and prices, let alone shadow prices) and behaviour (see, e.g.,
the measurement problems with respect to labour supply or with respect to the
allocation of time in general). In short, I am not much impressed by the
problems of conceptualization, nor by the measurement problems with respect
to preferences.

The measurement of preferences for the sake of improving our models
requires a change among both economists and social psychologists: they should
want to know more than they want to know now. In other words, economists should
be more interested in preferences than they find acceptable by the standards
of the perceived hard core of the neoclassical research programme. And social
psychologists should be more interested in improving economic and sociological
models, and not, as has been customary until now, to merely state that the
assumptions regarding preferences underlying these models contradict the
results of psychological research. We all know that; what we need to find out
is how we can make good use of this knowledge.

In most economic analyses of household decision making, it is assumed that both partners strive to maximize one joint final preference function. However, such a complete harmony of interests does not seem very plausible. Furthermore, an extension of the analysis to explain, for example, household dissolution, is precluded. It seems advisable to use a separate preference function for each partner. This raises a difficult yet interesting problem, namely the mutual adjustment of behaviour by both partners. The drawback of game-theoretical solutions is that they do not guarantee Pareto-optimal solutions (e.g. Kooreman, 1986). That is to say, they generally give rise to a state of equilibrium in which it is possible that one partner can improve his or her position, without hurting the other partner's position. This hardly seems plausible in a family context. On the other hand, the incorporation of Pareto-optimal solutions by viewing the household's final preference function as a convex combination of the final preference functions for both partners, yields only tractable, closed-form behavioural equations if a rather restricted specification is applied to the individual final preference functions, namely the Stone-Geary specification (cf. Kooreman, 1986; Grift and Siegers, 1989).

The application of the general rational-choice framework also involves the formulation of relevant restrictions: values and norms (partly related to attitudes of network members, including one's partner), expected and received support from network members (for example, for the realization of desires regarding a paid job, cf. Tazelaar and Sprengers, 1985), education, labour market situation, market prices (including wage rates), time, biological factors (Moors, 1974, pp. 119-129; Rosenzweig and Schultz, 1985), and so on. One must distinguish between actual restrictions, on the one hand, and perceived restrictions, on the other hand (see also Turchi, this volume). An illustration in point is the (expected) underestimation by young women of the increased probability of a miscarriage and the decreased probability of the realization of the desired family size when delaying pregnancy after the age of about 25 years (for more on these age-specific probabilities see Moors, 1986). Subjective assessments are also relevant where traditional economic variables are concerned, such as income (especially future income) and prices, as well as matters such as the availability of day-care facilities. Information strongly determines the discrepancy between perceived and actual values of variables. Information is in fact itself the outcome of a production process where time, market goods and the nature and size of social networks are the production factors.

A final step in applying the general rational-choice framework is to relate the preferences and restrictions to each other in a single explanatory model. The behavioural equations can be derived by maximizing the preference function, given the restrictions. To be able to test and estimate the model, it needs to be translated into an empirical estimation model that can be statistically analysed. The results of such analyses can then be used to improve the theoretical model.

Once the parameters of the theoretical models have been estimated, the models can be used for simulation analyses, for example, to evaluate policy measures. This can be illustrated by the following example. Let us assume that we want to know what the effect will be of tax or social security measures on the (timing of) male and female labour supply and their fertility. From the model estimation in the analytical phase, we know the parameters indicating the manner in which the wage rates of men and women as well as their social security benefits and non-wage income, if any, influence the (timing of) male and female labour supply and fertility. Changes in the tax or social security systems give rise to changes in the wage rates and in any social security benefits and non-wage income received; these changes can be calculated with knowledge of institutional regulations. Subsequently, we can determine the effect on the (timing of) male and female labour supply and fertility with the aid of the behavioural parameters estimated during the analytical phase (e.g. Bekkering *et al.*, 1986; Grift and Siegers, 1988).

14.5. Final comment

The present volume aims to show how the economic approach, which is itself a specification of the rational-choice approach, can be considerably more fertile than it has been in the past, because it offers an excellent theoretical framework for the construction of interdisciplinary theoretical models to explain human behaviour, including female labour supply and fertility.

Aigner, D. and G.C. Cain (1977), Statistical theories of discrimination in labor markets. *Industrial and Labor Relations Review*, 175-187.

Ajzen, I. (1985). From intentions to actions: a theory of planned behaviour. In: J. Kuhl and J. Beckmann (eds.), *Action-control: from cognition to behavior*. Heidelberg: Springer, 11-39.

Ajzen, I. and M. Fishbein (eds.) (1980), *Understanding attitudes and predicting social behaviour*. Englewood Cliffs: Prentice-Hall.

Ajzen, I. and T.J. Madden (1986), Prediction of goal-directed behaviour: attitudes, intentions, and perceived behavioral control. *Journal of Experimental Social Psychology*, 22, 453-474.

van den Akker, P.A.M. (1988), Between youth and adulthood: adolescents as unwed mothers. In: Moors and Schoorl (eds.), 323-338.

Almquist, E.M., S.S. Angrist and R. Mickelsen (1980), Women's career aspirations and achievements: college and seven years later. *Sociology of Work and Occupations*, 7, 376-384.

Amemiya, T. (1984), Tobit models: a survey. *Journal of Econometrics*, 24, 3-61.

Andorka, R. (1978), *Determinants of fertility in advanced societies*. London: Methuen and Co.

Ashenfelter, O. and R. Layard (eds.) (1986), *Handbook of labor economics*. Volume 1. Amsterdam: Elsevier.

Avioli, P.S. (1985). The labor-force participation of married mothers of infants. *Journal of Marriage and the Family*, 47, 739-745.

Bagozzi, R.P. (1981a), Attitudes, intentions, and behaviour: a test of some key hypotheses. *Journal of Personality and Social Psychology*, 41, 607-627.

Bagozzi, R.P. (1981b), An examination of the validity of two models of attitude. *Multivariate Behavioral Research*, 16, 323-359.

Bagozzi, R.P. (1984a), A prospectus for theory construction in marketing. *Journal of Marketing*, 48, 11-29.

Bagozzi, R.P. (1984b), Expectancy-value attitude models: an analysis of critical measurement issues. *International Journal of Research in Marketing*, 1, 295-310.

Bagozzi, R.P. (1985), Expectancy-value attitude models: an analysis of critical theoretical issues. *International Journal of Research in Marketing*, 2, 43-60.

Bagozzi, R.P. (1986), Attitude formation under the theory of reasoned action and a purposeful behaviour reformulation. *British Journal of Social Psychology*, 25, 95-107.

Bagozzi, R.P. (1989), An investigation of the role of affective and moral evaluations in the purposeful behaviour model of attitudes. *British Journal of Social Psychology*, 28, 97-113.

Bagozzi, R.P. (1990a), Multidimensional expectancy-value models in marketing research. Unpublished working paper, University of Michigan.

Bagozzi, R.P. (1990b), The role of arousal in the creation and control of the Halo effect. Unpublished working paper, University of Michigan.

Bagozzi, R.P. (1990c), An investigation of the effects of arousal on attitude structure. Unpublished working paper, University of Michigan.

Bagozzi, R.P. (1990d), On the neglect of volition in consumer research: a critique and proposal. Unpublished working paper, University of Michigan.

Bagozzi, R.P., J. Baumgartner and Y. Yi (1989), An investigation into the role of intentions as mediators of the attitude-behaviour relationship. *Journal of Economic Psychology*.

Bagozzi, R.P. and R.E. Burnkrant (1979), Attitude organization and the attitude-behaviour relationship. *Journal of Personality and Social Psychology*, 37, 913-929.

Bagozzi, R.P. and M.F. Van Loo (1978a), Fertility as consumption: theories from the behavioral sciences. *Journal of Consumer Research*, 4, 199-228.

Bagozzi, R.P. and M.F. Van Loo (1978b), Toward a general theory of fertility: a causal modeling approach. *Demography*, 15, 301-320.

Bagozzi, R.P. and M.F. Van Loo (1979), Rejoinder. *Journal of Consumer Research*, 5, 297-302.

Bagozzi, R.P. and M.F. Van Loo (1980), Decision-making and fertility: a theory of exchange in the family. In: Burch (ed.), 91-124.

Bagozzi, R.P. and M.F. Van Loo (1982), Fertility, labor force participation, and tastes: an economic psychology perspective. *Journal of Economic Psychology*, 2, 247-285.

Bagozzi, R.P. and M.F. Van Loo (1987), Individual and couple tastes for children: theoretical, methodological, and empirical issues. *Journal of Economic Psychology*, 8, 191-214.

Bagozzi, R.P. and M.F. Van Loo (1988), An investigation of the relationship between work and family size decisions over time. *Multivariate Behavioral Research*, 23, 3-34.

Bagozzi, R.P. and M.F. Van Loo (1990), Motivational and reasoned processes in the theory of consumer choice. Unpublished working paper, University of Michigan.

Bagozzi, R.P. and P.R. Warshaw (1990a), Trying to consume. *Journal of Consumer Research*, in press.

Bagozzi, R.P. and P.R. Warshaw (1990b), An examination of the etiology of the attitude-behaviour relation for goal-directed and mindless behavior. *Multivariate Behavioral Research*, in press.

Bagozzi, R.P. and Y. Yi (1989), The degree of intention formation as a moderator of the attitude-behaviour relation. *Social Psychology Quarterly*, 53, in press.

Bagozzi, R.P., Y. Yi and J. Baumgartner (1990), The level of effort required for behaviour as a moderator of the attitude-behaviour relation. *European Journal of Social Psychology*, 20, in press.

den Bandt, M.L. (1982), *Vrijwillig kinderloze vrouwen*. Deventer: Van Loghum Slaterus.

Bandura, A. (1977), Self-efficacy: toward a unifying theory of behavioural change. *Psychological Review*, 84, 191-215.

Bandura, A. (1982), Self-efficacy mechanism in human agency. *American Psychologist*, 37, 122-147.

Batra, R. and O. T. Ahtola (1987), The measurement and role of utilitarian and hedonic attitudes. Unpublished working paper, Columbia University.

Bauwens, S. and F. Deven (1989), *De kinderwens bevraagd: factoren die de intentie en de verwachte gevolgen bij de komst van een (volgend) kind beïnvloeden*. Werkdocument nr. 60. Brussel: CBGS.

Beck-Gernsheim, E. (1983), Vom 'Dasein für andere' zum Anspruch auf ein Stück 'eigenes Leben': Individualisierungsprozesse im weiblichen Lebenszusammenhang. *Soziale Welt*, 2, 307-337.

Becker, G.S. (1960), An economic analysis of fertility. In: National Bureau of Economic Research.

Becker, G.S. (1965), A theory of the allocation of time. *Economic Journal*, 75, 493-517.

Becker, G.S. (1975), The allocation of time over the life cycle. In: G.R. Ghez and G.S. Becker (eds.), *The allocation of time and goods over the life cycle*. New York: Columbia University Press, 83-132.

Becker, G.S. (1976), *The economic approach to human behavior*. Chicago: University of Chicago Press.

Becker, G.S. (1981), *A treatise on the family*. Cambridge: Harvard University Press.

Becker, G.S. (1988), Family economics and macro behavior. *American Economic Review*, 78, 3-13.

Becker, G.S. and R.J. Barro (1986), Altruism and the economic theory of fertility. In: Davis *et alii* (eds.), 69-76.

Becker, G.S. and H.G. Lewis (1973), On the interaction between the quantity and quality of children. *Journal of Political Economy*, 81, S279-S288.

Becker, G.S. and H.G. Lewis (1974), Interaction between quantity and quality of children. In: T.W. Schultz (ed.), 81-90.

Becker-Schmidt, R. (1981), Widersprüchliche Realität und Ambivalenz: Arbeitserfahrungen von Frauen in Fabrik und Familie. *Kölner Zeitschrift für Soziologie und Sozialpsychologie*, 32, 705-725.

Beckman, L.J. (1979), Fertility preferences and social exchange theory. *Journal of Applied Social Psychology*, 9, 147-169.

Beckman, L.J., R. Dizenberg, A.B. Forsythe, and T. Day (1983), A theoretical analysis of antecedents of young couples' fertility decisions and outcomes. *Demography*, 20, 519-533.

Bekkering, J., Y.K. Grift and J.J. Siegers (1986), *Belasting- en premieheffing en arbeidsmarktparticipatie door gehuwde vrouwen: een econometrische analyse*. 's-Gravenhage: Ministerie van Sociale Zaken en Werkgelegenheid.

Ben-Porath, Y. (1973), Labour force participation rates and the supply of labor. *Journal of Political Economy*, 81, 697-704.

Ben-Porath, Y. (1980), Transactional elements in a theory of fertility. In: Höhn and Mackensen (eds.), 49-58.

Berger, M. and L. Wright (1978), Divided allegiance: men, work, and family life. *Counseling Psychologist*, 4, 50-53.

Berger-Schmitt, R. (1986), Innerfamiliale Arbeitsteilung und ihre Determinanten. In: W. Glatzer and R. Berger-Schmitt (eds.), *Haushaltproduktion und Netzwerkhilfe*. Frankfurt: Campus, 105-140.

Berkowitz, L. and E. Walster (1976), *Advances in experimental social psychology*. Volume 9. New York: Academic Press.

Bernard, J. (1981), The good-provider role, its rise and fall. *American Psychologist*, 36, 43-48.

Bernhardt, E.M. (1986), Women's home attachment at first birth: the case of Sweden. *European Journal of Population*, 2, 5-29.

Bernhardt, E.M. (1987), *Labour force participation and childbearing: the impact of the first child on the economic activity of Swedish women*. Stockholm Research Reports in Demography, no. 41.

Bielby, W.T. and J.N. Baron (1986), Men and women at work: sex segregation and statistical discrimination. *American Journal of Sociology*, 91, 759-799.

Birg, H. (1987), *A biography approach to theoretical demography*. Materials of the Institute for Population Research and Social Policy, volume 23. Bielefeld: University of Bielefeld.

Birg, H., D. Filip and E.J. Flöthmann (1990), *Estimation and analysis of cohort and parity specific fertility data for post war West Germany*. Materials of the Institute for Population Research and Social Policy, volume 30. Bielefeld: University of Bielefeld (in German).

Birg, H. and E.J. Flöthmann (1990), Regionsspecifische Wechselwirkungen zwischen Migration und Fertilität im Lebenslauf. *Acta Demografica*, Deutsche Gesellschaft für Bevölkerungswissenschaft, Band 1, Heidelberg.

Birg, H., E.J. Flöthmann and I. Reiter (1989), Biographic analysis of the demographic characteristics of the life histories of men and women in regional labour market cohorts as clusters of birth cohorts. Paper prepared for the Symposium Life Histories and Generations, Netherlands Institute for Advanced Studies in the Humanities and Social Sciences, Wassenaar, June 1989.

Birg, H., E.J. Flöthmann and I. Reiter (forthcoming), *Biographische Theorie der demographischen Reproduktion - Demographische Verhaltensweisen regionaler Arbeitsmarktkohorten im biographischen Kontext*. Frankfurt: Campus.

Blackorby, C., G. Lady, D. Nissen and R.R. Russell (1970), Homothetic separability and consumer budgeting. *Econometrica*, 38, 468-472.

Blackorby, C., D. Primont and R.R. Russell (1978), *Duality, separability, and functional structure: theory and economic applications*. New York: North-Holland.

Blake, J. (1967), Income and reproductive motivation. *Population Studies*, 21, 185-206.

Blake, J. (1968), Are babies consumer durables ? Critique of the economic theory of reproductive motivation. *Population Studies*, 22, 5-25.

Blau, F.D. and M.A. Ferber (1986), *The economics of women, men and work*. Englewood Cliffs: Prentice-Hall.

Blaug, M. (1980), *The methodology of economics*. Cambridge: Cambridge University Press.

Boland, L.A. (1981), On the futility of criticizing the neoclassical maximization hypothesis. *American Economic Review*, 71, 1031-1036.

Bowen, W.G. and T.A. Finegan (1969), *The economics of labor force participation*. Princeton: Princeton University Press.

Bower, G.H. (1981), Mood and memory. *American Psychologist*, 36, 129-148.

Boyle, G.J. (1986), Higher-order factors in the differential emotions scale (DES-III). *Personality and Individual Differences*, 7, 305-310.

Brentano, L. (1872), *Die Arbeitergilden der Gegenwart, Zweiter Band: Zur Kritik der englischen Gewerkvereine*. Leipzig: Duncker und Humblot.

Brentano, L. (1909), *Die Malthus'sche Lehre und die Bevölkerungsbewegung der letzten Dezennien*. München: Abhandlungen der historischen Klasse der Königlich-Bayerischen Akademie der Wissenschaften, no. 24.

Brentano, L. (1910), The doctrine of Malthus and the increase of population during the last decades. *Economic Journal*, 20, 371-393.

Browning, M.J. (1982), Profit function representations for consumer preferences. Mimeo, Bristol University.

Browning, M.J., A. Deaton and M. Irish (1985), A profitable approach to labor supply and commodity demands over the life-cycle. *Econometrica*, 53, 503-543.

Büchl, W., L. von Rosenstiel and M. Stengel (1979), Wohnform und Kinderwunsch. *Zeitschrift für Bevölkerungswissenschaft*, 5, 185-198.

Bulatao, R.A. (1979), *Further evidence on the nature of the transition in the value of children*. Paper no. 60-B, East-West Population Institute, Honolulu.

Bulatao, R.A. (1981), Values and disvalues of children in successive childbearing decisions. *Demography*, 18, 1-26.

Bulatao, R.A. (1986), Does economic theory explain fertility ? *Family Planning Perspectives*, 18, 283-284.

Bulatao, R.A. and J.T. Fawcett (1981), Dynamic perspectives in the study of fertility decision-making: successive decisions within the fertility career. In: International Union for the Scientific Study of Population, *International Population Conference, Manila*. Volume 1. Liège: IUSSP, 433-449.

Burch, T.K. (ed.) (1980), *Demographic behaviour*. Boulder: Westview Press.

Burch, T.K. (1987), *Babel revisited: the role of ideas in explanations of human behaviour*. Discussion Paper 87-1, Population Studies Centre, University of Western Ontario.

Burnkrant, R.E. and R.J. Page (1988), The structure and antecedents of the normative and attitudinal components of Fishbein's theory of reasoned action. *Journal of Experimental Social Psychology*, 24, 66-87.

Busfield, J. and M. Paddon (1977), *Thinking about children. Sociology and fertility in post-war England*. Cambridge: Cambridge University Press.

Butz, W.P. and M.P. Ward (1979), The emergence of countercyclical U.S. fertility. *American Economic Review*, 69, 318-328.

Cain, G.G. and M.D. Dooley (1976), Estimation of a model of labor supply, fertility, and wages of married women. *Journal of Political Economy*, 84, S179-S199.

Caldwell, J.C. and A.G. Hill (1988), Recent developments using micro-approaches to demographic research. In: J.C. Caldwell, A.G. Hill and V.J. Hull (eds.), *Micro-approaches to demographic research*. London: Kegan Paul International, 1-24.

Calhoun, A.C. and T.J. Espenshade (1988), Childbearing and wives' foregone earnings. *Population Studies*, 42, 5-37.

Cameron, S. (1985), Towards a synthesis of economic and sociological theories of family labour supply. *Journal of Interdisciplinary Economics*, 1, 43-57.

Canlas, D.B. (1981), An economic analysis of marital fertility: some notes. *Philippine Economic Journal*, 20, 227-237.

Carliner, G., W.C. Robinson and N. Tomes (1984), Lifetime models of female labor supply, wage rates, and fertility. In: Schultz and Wolpin (eds.), 1-27.

Cigno, A. and J.F. Ermisch (1989), A microeconomic analysis of the timing of births. *European Economic Review*, 33, 737-760.

Clay, D.C. and J.J. Zuiches (1980), Reference groups and family size norms. *Population and Environment*, 3, 262-279.

Cochrane, S.H. (1979), *Fertility and education: what do we really know ?* World Bank Staff Occasional Papers No. 26. Baltimore: Johns Hopkins University Press.

Cole, J.R. and H. Zuckerman (1987), Marriage, motherhood and research performance in science. *Scientific American*, 119-125.

Coleman, S. (1983), The tempo of family formation. In: Plath (ed.), 183-214.

Coleman, J.S. (1990), *Foundations of social theory*. Cambridge: Harvard University Press.

Coombs, L.C. (1974), The measurement of family size preferences and subsequent fertility. *Demography*, 11, 587-611.

Corcoran, M., G.J. Duncan and M. Ponza (1983), Longitudinal analysis of white women's wages. *Journal of Human Resources*, 18, 497-520.

Cox, D.R. (1972), Regression models and lifetables. *Journal of the Royal Statistical Society*, Series B, 34, 187-220.

Cox, D.R. (1984), Panel estimates of the effects of career interruptions on the earnings of women. *Economic Inquiry*, 22, 386-403.

Cramer, J.C. (1980), Fertility and female employment: problems of causal direction. *American Sociological Review*, 45, 167-190.

Cramer, J.S. (1986), Het economisch onderzoek in de toekomst. In: H.M. Jolles, A.P. Plompen and H. Weijma (eds.), *Vijftien wetenschappen vijftien jaar verder*. 's-Gravenhage: Staatsuitgeverij, 37-52.

David, P.A. (1986), Comment on Becker and Barro's 'altruism and the economic theory of fertility'. In: Davis *et alii* (eds.), 77-86.

Davidson, A.R. and J.J. Jaccard (1975), Population psychology: a new look at an old problem. *Journal of Personality and Social Psychology*, 31, 1073-1082.

Davidson, A.R. and J.J. Jaccard (1979), Variables that moderate the attitude-behavior relation: results of a longitudinal survey. *Journal of Personality and Social Psychology*, 31, 1073-1082.

Davis, K. (1984), Wives and work: the sex role revolution and its consequences. *Population and Development Review*, 10, 397-417.

Davis, K., M.S. Bernstam and R. Ricardo-Campbell (eds.) (1986), *Below-replacement fertility in industrial societies: causes, consequences, policies*. A Supplement to Volume 12 of Population and Development Review.

Debusschere, R. and F. Deven (1981), *Het meten van de gezinsgroottevoorkeur*. CBGS Report 47. Brussel: CBGS.

Deven, F. (1979), The meanings of having children. In: R. Mackensen (ed.), *Seminarsbericht Empirische Untersuchungen zum generativen Verhalten*. Soziologischen Arbeitshefte no. 17, Berlin: Technische Universität, 54-68.

Deven, F. (1982), *Verwachtingen omtrent de komst van een (volgend) kind*. CBGS Report 57. Brussel: CBGS.

Deven, F. (1983), Parity-specific costs and benefits of childbearing: longitudinal data on decision-making by couples. In: R.L. Cliquet *et alii* (eds.), *Population and family in the low countries III*. NIDI/CBGS Publications Volume 10. Voorburg/Brussels: NIDI/CBGS, 109-121.

Deven, F. (1988), Characteristics, attitudes and expectations of voluntarily childless women, women intending to have children and mothers. In: H. Moors and J. Schoorl (eds.), 372-389.

Dooley, M.D. (1982), Labor supply and fertility of married women: an analysis with grouped and individual data from the 1970 U.S. Census. *Journal of Human Resources*, 17, 499-532.

Duesenberry, J.S. (1960), Comment on 'An economic analysis of fertility'. In: National Bureau for Economic Research, 231-234.

Easterlin, R.A. (1969), Towards a socioeconomic theory of fertility. In: S.J. Behrman, L. Corsa and R. Freedman (eds.), *Fertility and family planning: a world view*. Ann Arbor: University of Michigan Press, 127-156.

Easterlin, R.A. (1975), A framework for fertility analysis. *Studies in Family Planning*, 6, 54-63.

Easterlin, R.A. (1987), *Birth and fortune*. Chicago: University of Chicago Press.

Easterlin, R.A., R.A. Pollak and M.L. Wachter (1980), Toward a more general economic model of fertility determination: endogenous preferences and natural fertility. In: R.A. Easterlin (ed.), *Population and economic change in developing countries*. Chicago: University of Chicago Press, 81-149.

Eatwell, J., M. Milgate and P. Newman (1987) (eds.), *The new Palgrave: a dictionary of economics*. Volume 4. London: MacMillan, 287-297.

Edwards, W. (1961), Behavioural decision theory. *Annual Review of Psychology*, 12, 473-498.

Elchardus, M. (1984), Life cycle and life course: the scheduling and temporal integration of life. In: S. Feld and R. Lesthaeghe (eds.), *Population and social outlook*. Brussels: Koning Boudewijn Stichting, 251-267.

England, P. (1982), The failure of human capital theory to explain occupational sex segregation. *Journal of Human Resources*, 17, 358-370.

England, P. (1984), Wage appreciation and depreciation: a test of neoclassical economic explanations of occupational sex segregation. *Social Forces*, 62, 726-749.

Erikson, E.H. (1980), *Identity and the life cycle*. New York: Norton and Company.

Ermisch, J.F. (1989), Purchased child care, optimal family size and mothers' employment: theory and econometric analysis. *Journal of Population Economics*, 2, 79-102.

Etzioni, A. (1967), Mixed scanning: a third approach to decision making. *Public Administration Review*, 27, 385-292.

Even, W.E. (1982), Career interruptions following childbirth. *Journal of Labor Economics*, 5, 255-277.

Everitt, A.V. (1982), The genetic clock-hormone theory of aging. In: S. Preston (ed.), *Biological and social aspects of mortality and the length of life*. Liège: Ordina, 279-300.

Eysenck, H.J. (1986), Models and paradigms in personality research. In: A. Angleiter, A. Furnham and G. van Heck (eds.), *Personality psychology in Europe, Volume 2: Current trends and controversies*. Lisse: Swets and Zeitlinger, 213-223.

Falbo, T. and H.A. Becker (1980), The Fishbein model: triumphs, problems and prospects. In: Burch (ed.), 125-140.

Fawcett, J.T. and F. Arnold (1973), The value of children: theory and method. *Representative Research in Social Psychology*, 4, 23-36.

Fishbein, M. (1982), Toward an understanding of family planning behaviors. *Journal of Applied Social Psychology*, 2, 214-227.

Fishbein, M. and I. Ajzen (1975), *Belief, attitude, intention and behavior: an introduction to theory and research*. Reading: Addison-Wesley.

Fleisher, B.M. and G.F. Rhodes Jr. (1979), Fertility, women's wage rates, and labor supply. *American Economic Review*, 69, 14-24.

Fried, E.S., S.L. Hofferth and J.R. Udry (1980), Parity specific and two-sex utility models of reproductive intentions. *Demography*, 17, 1-12.

Fried, E.S. and J.R. Udry (1980), Normative pressures on fertility planning. *Population and Environment*, 3, 199-209.

Fuchs, V.R. (1983), *How we live: an economic perspective on Americans from birth to death*. Cambridge: Harvard University Press.

Fuchs, V.R. (1986), *The health economy*. Cambridge: Harvard University Press.

Fürstenberg, F. and J. Mörth (1979), Religionssoziologie. In: *Handbuch der empirischen Sozialforschung*. Band 14. Stuttgart: Enke.

van Geert, P. (1986), The concept of development. In: P. van Geert (ed.), *Theory building in developmental psychology*. Amsterdam: North Holland, 3-50.

Georgescu-Roegen, N. (1970), The economics of production. *American Economic Review*, 60, 1-9.

Gorman, W.M. (1959), Separable utility and aggregation. *Econometrica*, 27, 469-481.

Gorman, W.M. (1987), Separability. In: J. Eatwell *et alii* (eds.), 305-312.

Greene, W.H. and A.O. Quester (1982), Divorce risk and wives' labor supply behavior. *Social Science Quarterly*, 63, 16-27.

Grift, Y.K. and J.J. Siegers (1988), Supply determinants of part-time work of Dutch married women: the influence of taxes and social premiums. Paper presented at the Second Annual Meeting of the European Society for Population Economics, Mannheim, June 23-25, 1988.

Grift, Y.K. and J.J. Siegers (1989), Estimating an individual utility labour supply model with a family budget constraint and with Pareto optimal outcomes. Paper presented at the Third Annual Meeting of the European Society for Population Economics, Bouray-sur-Juine, June 8-10, 1989.

Gronau, R. (1974), Wage comparisons - a selectivity bias. *Journal of Political Economy*, 82, 1119-1143.

Groot, L.F.M., J.J. Schippers and J.J. Siegers (1988), The effect of interruptions and part-time work on women' wage rate: a test of the variable-intensity model. *De Economist*, 136, 220-238.

Groot, L.F.M., J.J. Schippers and J.J. Siegers (forthcoming), The effect of unemployment, temporary withdrawals and part-time work on workers' wage rates. *European Sociological Review*.

Hass, P.H. (1974), Wanted and unwanted pregnancies: a fertility decision-making model. *Journal of Social Issues*, 30, 125-165.

Hausman, J.A. (1979), Individual discount rates and the purchase and utilization of energy-using durables. *Bell Journal of Economics*, 10, 33-54.

Heckman, J.J. (1974a), Life cycle consumption and labor supply: an explanation of the relationship between income and consumption over the life cycle. *American Economic Review*, 64, 188-194.

Heckman, J.J. (1974b), Shadow prices, market wages and labor supply. *Econometrica*, 42, 679-694.

Heckman, J.J. (1976a), The common structure of statistical models of truncation, sample selection and limited dependent variables and a simple estimator for such models. *Annals of Economic and Social Measurement*, 5, 475-492.

Heckman, J.J. (1976b), A life-cycle model of earnings, learning, and consumption. *Journal of Political Economy*, 84, S11-S44.

Heckman, J.J. (1977), Sample selection bias as a specification error. *Econometrica*, 47, 153-162.

Heckman, J.J. (1980), Sample selection bias as a specification error. In: J. Smith (ed.), *Female labor supply*. Princeton: Princeton University Press, 206-248.

Heckman, J.J. (1981), Heterogeneity and state dependence. In: S. Rosen (ed.), *Studies in labor markets*. Chicago: University of Chicago Press, 91-139.

Heckman, J.J. (1987), Selection bias and self-selection. In: J. Eatwell *et alii* (eds.), 287-297.

Heckman, J.J., V.J. Hotz and J. Walker (1985), New evidence on the timing and spacing of births. *American Economic Review*, 75, 179-184.

Heckman, J.J. and T.E. MaCurdy (1980), A life cycle model of female labour supply. *Review of Economic Studies*, 47, 47-74.

Heckman, J.J. and T.E. MaCurdy (1982), Corrigendum on a life cycle model of female labour supply. *Review of Economic Studies*, 49, 659-660.

Held, T. (1986), Institutionalization and de-institutionalization of the life course. *Human Development*, 29, 157-162.

Helson, H. (1964), *Adaption-level theory*. New York: Harper and Row.

Hill, C.R. and F.P. Stafford (1985a), Lifetime fertility, child care, and labor supply. In: F.T. Juster *et alii* (eds.), 471-492.

Hill, C.R. and F.P. Stafford (1985b), Parental care of children: time diary estimates of quantity, predictability, and variety. In: F.T. Juster *et alii* (eds.), 415-437.

Hiller, D.V. and J. Dyehouse (1987), A case for banishing dual-career marriages from the research literature. *Journal of Marriage and the Family*, 49, 787-795.

Hirsch, F. (1978), *Social limits to growth*. Cambridge: Harvard University Press.

Hoem, B. and J.M. Hoem (1989), The impact of women's employment on second and third births in modern Sweden. *Population Studies*, 43, 47-67.

Hoffman, A. (1978), The value of children to parents in the United States. *Journal of Population*, 1, 91-131.

Höhn, C. and R. Mackensen (1980) (eds.), *Determinants of fertility trends: theories re-examined*. Liège: Ordina Editions.

Holden, K.C. (1983), Changing employment patterns of women. In: Plath (ed.), 36-46.

Hotz, V.J. and R.A. Miller (1988), An empirical analysis of life cycle fertility and female labor supply. *Econometrica*, 56, 91-118.

Ickes, W. (1985), Introduction. In: W. Ickes (ed.), *Compatible and incompatible relationships*. New York: Springer Verlag, 1-7.

Impens, K. (1987), De impact van werkloosheid bij vrouwen op de vruchtbaarheid in Vlaanderen. *Bevolking en Gezin*, 3, 73-98.

Inglehart, R. (1977), *The silent revolution*. Princeton.

Inglehart, R. (1979), *Married women and work*. Toronto.

Inglehart, R. (1989), *Kultureller Umbruch*. Frankfurt: Campus.

Janis, I.L. and L. Mann (1977), *Decision making: a psychological analysis of conflict, choice and commitment*. New York: Free Press.

Jansweijer, R.M.A., E.M. Pot, H.J. Groenendijk and H.M. Langeveld (1988), *Haalbaar en betaalbaar: arbeid en kinderzorg na 1990*. Rotterdam: Erasmus Universiteit, sectie Vrouwenstudies.

Johnson, M.D. and C.P. Puto (1988), A review of consumer judgment and choice. In: M.J. Houston (ed.), *Review of marketing 1987*. Chicago: American Marketing Association.

Johnson, T.R. and J.H. Pencavel (1984), Dynamic hours of work functions for husbands, wives, and single females. *Econometrica*, 52, 363-389.

Johnson, W.R. and J. Skinner (1985), Labor supply and marital se-paration. Paper presented at the Economic Demography Workshop, Population Association of America.

Jones, E.B. and J.E. Long (1979), Part-week work and human capital investment by married women. *Journal of Human Resources*, 14, 563-578.

Joshi, H. (1988), *Changing roles of women in the British labour market and the family*. Discussion Paper in Economics 88/13, Birkbeck College, University of London.

Jürgens, H.W. and K. Pohl (1975), *Kinderzahl - Wunsch und Wirklichkeit*. Stuttgart.

Juster, F.T. and F.P. Stafford (eds.) (1985), *Time, goods, and well-being*. Ann Arbor: University of Michigan.

van de Kaa, D.J. (1988), *The second demographic transition revisited: theories and expectations*. Werkstukken no. 109, Planologisch Demografisch Instituut, Universiteit van Amsterdam.

van de Kaa, D.J. and H.G. Moors (1982), Social status, social structure and fertility: a critical review with special reflections on the Netherlands. In: Département de Démographie de l'Université de Louvain (ed.), *Population et structures sociales*, Liège: Ordina, 107-127.

Kahn-Hut, R., A.K. Daniels and R. Colvard (1982), *Women and work*. New York.

Kapteyn, A. (ed.) (1987), *Demografische veranderingen en economische ontwikkelingen*. Preadviezen voor de Koninklijke Vereniging voor de Staathuishoudkunde. Leiden: Stenfert Kroese.

Klages, H. and P. Kmieciak (1979), *Wertwandel und gesellschaftlicher Wandel*. Frankfurt.

Keeley, M.C. (1975), A comment on 'An interpretation of the economic theory of fertility'. *Journal of Economic Literature*, 13, 467-468.

Kenny, D.A. and C.M. Judd (1984), Estimating the nonlinear and interactive effects of latent variables. *Psychological Bulletin*, 96, 201-210.

Keyfitz, N. (1977), *Applied mathematical demography*. New York: Wiley.

Killingsworth, M.R. (1983), *Labor supply*. Cambridge: Cambridge University Press.

Killingsworth, M.R. and J.J. Heckman (1986), Female labor supply: a survey. In: Ashenfelter and Layard (eds.), 103-204.

Kinsella, R.P. (1975), A note on the new home economics. *International Journal of Social Economics*, 2, 249-257.

Kiser, C.V. (1979), Comments on 'Fertility as consumption: theories from the behavioral sciences'. *Journal of Consumer Research*, 5, 284-287.

Kiser, C.V. and P.K. Whelpton (1953), Resume of the Indianapolis study of social and psychological factors affecting fertility. *Population Studies*, 7, 95-110.

Kiser, C.V. and P.K. Whelpton (1958), Social and psychological factors affecting fertility. *Milbank Memorial Fund Quarterly*, 36, 282-329.

Kleining, G. and H. Moore (1968), Soziale Selbsteinstufung: ein Instrument zur Messung sozialer Schichten. *Kölner Zeitschrift für Soziologie und Sozialpsychologie*, 20, 273-292.

Klijzing, E., J. Siegers, N. Keilman and L. Groot (1988), Static versus dynamic analysis of the interaction between female labour force participation and fertility. *European Journal of Population*, 4, 97-116.

Kooreman, P. (1986), *Essays on the microeconomic analysis of household behaviour*. PhD-dissertation, Tilburg: Katholieke Universiteit Brabant.

Korpi, T. (1989), *Entry into employment after first birth: a reexamination of the transitions to full-time and part-time employment among Swedish mothers*. Stockholm Research Reports in Demography, no 53.

Lakatos, I. (1970), Falsification and the methodology of scientific research programmes. In: I. Lakatos and A. Musgrave (eds.), *Criticism and the growth of knowledge*. Cambridge: Cambridge University Press.

Lancaster, K.J. (1966), A new approach to consumer theory. *Journal of Political Economy*, 74, 132-157.

Larsson, L.G. (1977), Economic models of household behavior. In: Å. Andersson and I. Holmberg (eds.), *Demographic, economic and social interaction*, Cambridge: Ballinger, 119-145.

Latsis, S.J. (1976), A research programme in economics. In: S.J. Latsis (ed.), *Method and appraisal in economics*. Cambridge: Cambridge University Press, 1-41.

Lazear, E.P. and R.T. Michael (1988), *Allocation of income within the household*. Chicago: University of Chicago Press.

Lehr, U. (1984), Stereotypie und Wandlung der Geschlechtsrollen. In: A. Heigl-Evers (ed.), *Sozialpsychologie*. Weinheim: Beltz.

Lehrer, E. and M. Nerlove (1986), Female labor force behavior and fertility in the United States. *Annual Review of Sociology*, 12, 181-204.

Leibenstein, H. (1957), *Economic backwardness and economic growth: studies in the theory of economic development*. New York: Wiley.

Leibenstein, H. (1974), An interpretation of the economic theory of fertility: promising path or blind alley ? *Journal of Economic Literature*, 12, 457-479.

Leibenstein, H. (1979), Comments on 'Fertility as consumption: theories from the behavioral sciences'. *Journal of Consumer Research*, 5, 287-290.

Leibenstein, H. (1980), Relaxing the maximization assumption in the economic theory of fertility. In: Höhn and Mackensen (eds.), 35-48.

Lerner, R.M. and M.B. Kauffman (1985), The concept of development in contextualism. *Developmental Review*, 5, 309-333.

Levinson, D.J. *et alii* (1978), *The seasons of a man's life*. New York: Ballantine Books.

Levinson, D.J. and W.L. Gooden (1985), The life cycle. In: N.I. Kaplan and B.J. Sadock (eds.), *Comprehensive textbook of psychiatry*. Baltimore: Williams and Wilkins, 1-13.

Lewis, H.G. (1967), On income and substitution effects in labor force participation. Unpublished manuscript, University of Chicago.

Lindenberg, S. (1982), Sharing groups: theory and suggested applications, *Journal of Mathematical Sociology*, 9, 33-62.

Lindenberg, S. (1984a), Normen und die Allokation sozialer Wertschätzung. In: H. Todt (ed.), *Normengeleitetes Verhalten in den Sozialwissenschaften*. Berlin: Duncker und Humblot, 169-191.

Lindenberg, S. (1984b), Preference versus constraints. *Journal of Institutional and Theoretical Economics* (ZgS), 140, 96-103.

Lindenberg, S. (1985), An assessment of the new political economy: its potential for the social sciences and for sociology in particular. *Sociological Theory*, 3, 99-114.

Lindenberg, S. (1986), The paradox of privatization in consumption. In: A. Diekmann and P. Mitter (eds.), *Paradoxial effects of social behavior*. Heidelberg/Wien: Physica-Verlag, 297-310.

Lindenberg, S. (1988), Contractual relations and weak solidarity: the behavioral basis of restraints on gain-maximization. *Journal of Institutional and Theoretical Economics* (ZgS), 144, 39-58.

Lindenberg, S. (1989), Choice and culture: the Behavioral basis of cultural impact on transactions. In: H. Haferkamp (ed.), *Social structure and culture*. Berlin: de Gruyter.

Liska, A.E. (1984), A critical examination of the causal structure of the Fishbein/Ajzen attitude-behavior model. *Social Psychology Quarterly*, 47, 61-74.

MaCurdy, T. (1977), Labor supply decisions over the life cycle. Unpublished manuscript, University of Chicago.

MaCurdy, T. (1978), *Two essays on the life cycle*. PhD-thesis, University of Chicago.

Marini, M.M. and B. Singer (1988), Causality in social sciences. *Sociological methodology*, 18, 347-409.

Maslow, A.H. (1954), *Motivation and personality*. New York: Harper and Row.

Maslow, A.H. (1973), A theory of human motivation. *Psychological Review*, 50, 370-396.

McClelland, G.H. (1983). Family-size desires as measures of demand. In: R.A. Bulatao and R.D. Lee (eds.), *Determinants of fertility in developing countries. Volume 1: Supply and Demand for Children*. New York: Academic Press, 288-343.

McKenry, P., S.J. Price, P.B. Gordon and N.M. Rudd (1986), Characteristics of husband's family work and wives' labor force involvement. In: R. Lewis and R.E. Salt (eds.), *Men in Families*. Beverly Hills: Sage, 73-83.

Michael, R.T. and G.S. Becker. (1973), On the new theory of consumer behavior. *Swedish Journal of Economics*, 75, 378-396.

Miller, P.H. (1983), *Theories of developmental psychology*. San Francisco: Freemand and Company.

Miller, W.B. (1980), *The psychology of reproduction*. Springfield: National Technical Information Service.

Miller, W.B. (1986), Proception: an important fertility behavior. *Demography*, 23, 579-594.

Mincer, J. (1962), Labor force participation of married women: a study of labor supply. In: National Bureau of Economic Research, *Aspects of labor economics*. Princeton: Princeton University Press, 63-97.

Mincer, J. (1963), Market prices, opportunity costs and income effects. In: C.F. Christ (ed.), *Measurement in economics*. Stanford, 67-82.

Mincer, J. and H. Ofek (1982), Interrupted work careers: depreciation and restoration of human capital. *Journal of Human Resources*, 17, 3-24.

Mincer, J. and S. Polachek (1974), Family investments in human capital: earnings of women. In: Schultz (ed.), 397-429.

Mincer, J. and S. Polachek (1978), Women's earnings reexamined. *Journal of Human Resources*, 13, 118-134.

Mischel, W. (1977), On the future of personality measurement. *American Psychologist*, 32, 246-254.

Mitchell, W.C. (1912), The backward art of spending money. *American Economic Review*, 2, 269-281.

Moffitt, R.A. (1984a). Optimal life-cycle profiles of fertility and labor supply. In: Schultz and Wolpin (eds.), 29-50.

Moffitt, R.A. (1984b), Profiles of fertility, labour supply and wages of married women: a complete life cycle model. *Review of Economic Studies*, 51, 263-278.

Mol, P.W., J.C. van Ours and J.J.M. Theeuwes (1988), *Honderd jaar gehuwde vrouwen op de arbeidsmarkt*. OSA-werkdocument nr. 4. 's-Gravenhage: Organisatie voor Strategisch Arbeidsmarktonderzoek.

Mombert, P. (1907), *Studien zur Bevölkerungsbewegung in Deutschland*. Karlsruhe: Braun.

Moore-Ede, M.C., F.M. Sulzman and C.A. Fuller (1982), *The clocks that time us: physiology of the circadian timing system*. Cambridge: Harvard University Press.

Moors, H.G. (1974), *Child spacing and family size in the Netherlands*. Leiden: Stenfert Kroese.

Moors, H.G. (1986), Moeder worden op oudere leeftijd: een nieuwe trend ? *Demos*, 2, 9-12.

Moors, H. and J. Schoorl (eds.) (1988), *Lifestyles, contraception and parenthood*. The Hague/Brussels: NIDI/CBGS.

Mott, F.L. (1972), Fertility, life-cycle stage and female labor force participation in Rhode Island: a retrospective view. *Demography*, 9, 173-185.

Mott, F.L. and D. Shapiro (1983), Complementarity of work and fertility among young American mothers. *Population Studies*, 37, 239-252.

Mroz, T.A. (1987), The sensitivity of an empirical model of married women's hours of work to economic and statistical assumptions. *Econometrica*, 55, 765-799.

Muth, R.F. (1966), Household production and economic demand functions. *Econometrica*, 34, 699-708.

Nakamura, A. and M. Nakamura (1981a), A comparison of the labor force behavior of married women in the United States and Canada, with special attention to the impact of income taxes. *Econometrica*, 49, 451-489.

Nakamura, A. and M. Nakamura (1981b), On the relationships among several specification error tests presented by Durbin, Wu and Hausman. *Econometrica*, 49, 1583-1588.

Nakamura, A. and M. Nakamura (1983), Part-time and full-time work behaviour of married women: a model with a doubly truncated dependent variable. *Canadian Journal of Economics*, 16, 229-257.

Nakamura, A. and M. Nakamura (1984), On the roles of child status and marital status variables in models of the labor force behavior of married women. Paper presented at the Econometric Society Meeting in Dallas, December 1984.

Nakamura, A. and M. Nakamura (1985a), Dynamic models of the labor force behavior of married women which can be estimated using limited amounts of past information. *Journal of Econometrics*, 27, 273-298.

Nakamura, A. and M. Nakamura (1985b), *The second paycheck: a socioeconomic analysis of earnings*. New York: Academic Press.

Nakamura, A. and M. Nakamura (1985c), On the performance of tests by Wu and by Hausman for detecting the ordinary least squares bias problem. *Journal of Econometrics*, 29, 213-227.

Nakamura, A. and M. Nakamura (1987), Theories and evidence concerning the impacts of children on female labor supply. Paper presented at the Canadian Economic Association Meeting in Hamilton, Ontario, June 1987.

Nakamura, A. and M. Nakamura (1989), Selection bias: more than a female phenomenon. In: B. Raj (ed.), *Advances in econometrics and modelling*. Deventer: Kluwer, 143-158.

Nakamura, M., A. Nakamura and D. Cullen (1979), Job opportunities, the offered wage, and the labor supply of married women. *American Economic Review*, 69, 787-805.

Namboodiri, N.K. (1972a), Integrative potential of a fertility model: an analytical test. *Population Studies*, 26, 465-485.

Namboodiri, N.K. (1972b), Some observations on the economic framework for fertility analysis. *Population Studies*, 26, 185-206.

Namboodiri, N.K. (1974), Which couples at given parities expect to have additional births ? An exercise in discriminant analysis. *Demography*, 11, 45-56.

Namboodiri, N.K. (1975), Review of: T.W. Schultz (ed.), Economics of the family: marriage, children and human capital. *Demography*, 12, 561-569.

Namboodiri, N.K. (1978), On fertility analysis. Where sociologists, economists, and biologists meet. In: J.M. Yinger and S.J. Cutler (eds.), *Major social issues: a multidisciplinary view*. New York: Free Press, 295-309.

Namboodiri, N.K. (1979), Fertility as consumption: theories from the behavioral sciences: Comment. *Journal of Consumer Research*, 5, 290-292.

Namboodiri, N.K. (1980), A look at fertility model building from different perspectives. In: Burch (ed.), 71-90.

Namboodiri, N.K. (1983), Sequential fertility decision making and the life course. In: R.A. Bulatao and R.D. Lee (eds.), *Determinants of fertility in developing countries. Volume 2: Fertility regulation and institutional influences*. New York: Academic Press, 444-472.

National Bureau for Economic Research (1960), *Demographic and economic change in developed countries*. Princeton: Princeton University Press.

Nerdinger, F.W. (1984), Stabilität, Zentralität und Verhaltensrelevanz von Werten. *Problem und Entscheidung*, 26, 86-110.

Nerdinger, F.W. *et alii* (1984), Kinderwunsch und generatives Verhalten: ausgewählte Ergebnisse einer Längsschnittstudie an jungen Ehepaaren. *Zeitschrift für experimentelle und angewandte Psychologie*, 31, 464-482.

Ni Bhrolchain, M. (1986a), Women's paid work and the timing of births: longitudinal evidence. *European Journal of Population*, 2, 43-70.

Ni Bhrolchain, M. (1986b), The interpretation and role of work-associated accelerated childbearing in post-war Britain. *European Journal of Population*, 2, 135-154.

Niphuis-Nell, M. (1981), *Motivatie voor ouderschap*. Deventer: Van Loghum Slaterus.

Niphuis-Nell, M. and H.G. Moors (1979), *De constructie van meetinstrumenten in het NOVOM-1975*. Intern Rapport no. 16. Voorburg: NIDI.

Noelle-Neumman, E. and B. Strümpel (1984), *Macht Arbeit krank, macht Arbeit glücklich ?* München: Piper.

Oberschall, A. and E.M. Leifer (1986), Efficiency and social institutions: uses and misuses of economic reasoning in sociology. *Annual Review of Sociology*, 12, 233-254.

Okun, B. (1960), Comment. In: National Bureau for Economic Research, 235-240.

Opp, K.D. (1985a), Sociology and economic man. *Journal of Institutional and Theoretical Economics* (ZgS), 141, 213-243.

Opp, K.D. (1985b), *Die Entstehung sozialer Normen*. Tübingen: Mohr Siebeck.

Ory, M.G. (1978), The decision to parent or not: normative and structural components. *Journal of Marriage and the Family*, 40, 531-539.

Paarsch, H. (1984), A Monte Carlo comparison of estimators for censored regression models. *Journal of Econometrics*, 24, 197-214.

Parsons, T. (1937/1968), *The structure of social action*. Paperback edition. New York: Free Press.

Parsons, T. (1954), The incest taboo in relation to social structure and the socialization of the child. *The Britisch Journal of Sociology*, 5, 2.

Pauwels, K., M. de Wachter, L. Deschamps and W. van Dongen (1987), The labour force participation by young women with a family: a lasting commitment. In: H.G. Moors *et alii* (eds.), *Population and family in the low countries V*. The Hague/Brussels: NIDI/CBGS, 1-13.

Pencavel, J. (1986), Labor supply of men: a survey. In: Ashenfelter and Layard (eds.), 3-102.

Perlman, M. (1975), Review of: T.W. Schultz (ed.), Economics of the family: marriage, children and human capital. *Demography*, 12, 549-556.

Phelps, E. (1972), The statistical theory of racism and sexism. *American Economic Review*, 62, 659-661.

Picot, G. (1987), Modelling the lifetime employment patterns of Canadians. In: Proceedings of conference on the family in crisis.

Plath, D.W. (ed.) (1983), *Work and lifecourse in Japan*. Albany: State University of New York Press.

Polachek, S. (1976), Occupational segregation: an alternative hypothesis. *Journal of Contemporary Business*, 5, 1-12.

Polachek, S. (1979), Occupational segregation among women: theory, evidence, and a prognosis. In: C. Lloyd, E. Andrews and C. Gilroy (eds.), *Women in the labor market*, New York: Columbia University Press, 137-157.

Polachek, S. (1981), Occupational self-selection: a human capital approach to sex differences in occupational structure. *Review of Economics and Statistics*, 58, 60-69.

Population Studies Centre, University of Western Ontario (1988), *Canadian fertility survey, 1984: public use micro-data documentation*.

Presser, H.B. (1986), Shift work among American women and child care. *Journal of Marriage and the Family*, 48, 551-564.

Presser, H.B. (1988), Shift work and child care among young dual-earner American parents. *Journal of Marriage and the Family*, 50, 133-148.

Regan, M.C. and H.E. Roland (1985), Rearranging family and career priorities: professional women and men of the eighties. *Journal of Marriage and the Family*, 47, 985-992.

Reid, M.G. (1934), *Economics of household production*. New York: Wiley.

Robbins, L. (1930), On the elasticity of demand for income in terms of effort. *Economica*, 29, 123-129.

Robinson, W.C. (1987), The time cost of children and other household production. *Population Studies*, 41, 313-323.

Robinson, W.C. and N. Tomes (1985), More on the labour supply of Canadian women. *Canadian Journal of Economics*, 18, 156-163.

Rogers, B. (1980), *The domestication of women*. London: Kogan Page.

von Rosenstiel, L. (1987), *Grundlagen der Organisationspsychologie*. Stuttgart: Poeschel.

von Rosenstiel, L. *et alii* (1986), *Einführung in die Bevölkerungspsychologie*. Darmstadt: Wissenschaftliche Buchgesellschaft.

von Rosenstiel, L., G. Oppitz and M. Stengel (1982), Motivation of reproductive behaviour: a theoretical concept and its application. In: Höhn and Mackensen (eds.), 79-93.

von Rosenstiel, L. and M. Stengel (1987), *Identifikationskrise ? Zum Engagement in betrieblichen Führungspositionen*. Bern: Huber.

Rosenzweig, M.R. and T.P. Schultz (1985), The demand for and supply of births: fertility and its life cycle consequences. *American Economic Review*, 75, 992-1015.

Rosenzweig, M.R. and K.I. Wolpin (1980), Life-cycle labor supply and fertility: causal inferences from household models. *Journal of Political Economy*, 88, 328-348.

Roth, J.A. (1963), *Timetables*. Indianapolis: Bobbs-Merrill.

Roth, J.A. (1983), Timetables and the lifecourse in post-industrial society. In: Plath (ed.), 248-259.

Rozendal, P.J., H.G. Moors and F.L. Leeuw (1985), *Het bevolkingsvraagstuk in de jaren '80*. Voorburg: NIDI.

Rubin, Z. (1973), *Liking and Loving*. New York: Holt, Rinehart and Winston.

Runyan, W.M. (1984), *Life histories and psychobiography: explorations in theory and method*. New York: Oxford University Press.

Russell, J.A. (1979), Affective space is bipolar. *Journal of Personality and Social Psychology*, 37, 345-356.

Ryder, N.B. (1965), The cohort as a concept in the study of social change. *American Sociological Review*, 30, 843-861.

Ryder, N.B. (1973). Comment. *Journal of Political Economy*, 81, S65-S69.

Salmon, W.C. (1984), *Scientific explanation and the causal structure of the world*. Princeton: Princeton University Press.

Sandell, S.H. and D. Shapiro (1978), Theory of human capital and the earnings of women: a reexamination of the evidence. *Journal of Human Resources*, 13, 103-117.

Sandell, S.H. and D. Shapiro (1980), Work expectations, human capital accumulation, and the wages of young women. *Journal of Human Resources*, 15, 335-353.

Sandy, R. (1977), *Two essays in the history of short-run labor supply theory*. PhD-dissertation, Michigan State University, Ann Arbor.

Scanzoni, J.H. (1975), *Sex roles, life styles, and childbearing*. New York: Free Press.

Scanzoni, J.H. (1978), *Sex roles, women's work and navital conflict*. Toronto.

Scanzoni, J.H. (1979), Comments on 'Fertility as consumption: theories from the behavioral sciences'. *Journal of Consumer Research*, 5, 292-293.

Schubnell, H. (1973), *Der Geburtenrückgang in der BRD - Die Entwicklung der Erwerbstätigkeit von Frauen und Müttern*. Stuttgart.

Schultz, T.P. (1976), Determinants of fertility: a micro-economic model of choice. In: A.J. Coale (ed.), *Economic factors in population growth*. New York: Wiley, 89-124.

Schultz, T.P. (1978), The influence of fertility on labor supply of married women: simultaneous equation estimates. In: R. Ehrenky (ed.), *Research in labor economics*. Volume 2. Greenwich: JAI Press, 273-351.

Schultz, T.P. (1981), *Economics of population*. Reading: Addison-Wesley.

Schultz, T.P. and K.I. Wolpin (eds.) (1984), *Research in population economics*. Volume 5. Greenwich: JAI Press.

Schultz, T.W. (ed.) (1974), *Economics of the family: marriage, children and human capital*. Chicago: University of Chicago Press.

Schwarz, K. (1981), Erwerbstätigkeit der Frauen und Kinderzahl. *Zeitschrift für Bevölkerungswissenschaft*, 7, 59-87.

Sen, A. (1973), Behaviour and the concept of preference. *Economica*, 40, 241-259.

Shaw, L.B. (1983), Causes of irregular employment patterns. In: L.B. Shaw (ed.), *Unplanned careers: the working lives of middle-aged women*. Lexington: Lexington Books, 45-59.

Siegers, J.J. (1985), *Arbeidsaanbod en kindertal: een micro-economische analyse*. PhD-thesis, Groningen University.

Siegers, J.J. (1987), Economische verklaringen van het kindertal. In: Kapteyn (ed.), 89-124.

Siegers, J.J. (1990), Towards the construction of interdisciplinary theoretical models to explain demographic behaviour. In: C.A. Hazeu and G.A.B. Frinking (eds.), *Emerging issues in demographic research*. Amsterdam: Elsevier, 181-196.

Simon, H.A. (1978), Rationality as process and product of thought. *American Economic Review*, 68, 1-16.

Simon, H.A. (1979), The meaning of causal ordering. In: R.K. Merton, J.S. Coleman and P.H. Rossi (eds.), *Qualitative and quantitative social research*. London: Free Press, 65-81.

Sinclair, D. (1985), *Human growth after birth*. Fourth edition. Oxford: Oxford University Press.

Skeen, P., L.P. Pauio, B.E. Robinson and J.E. Deal (1989), Mothers working outside of the home: attitudes of fathers and mothers in three cultures. In: E.B. Goldsmith (ed.), *Work and family*. Newbury Park: Sage, 373-382.

Smith, A. (1776/1970), *An inquiry into the nature and causes of the wealth of nations*. London: Aldine Press.

Smith, J.B. and M. Stelcner (1988), Labour supply of married women in Canada, 1980. *Canadian Journal of Economics*, 21, 857-870.

Smith-Lovin, L. and A.R. Tickamyer (1978), Nonrecursive models of labor force participation, fertility behaviour, and sex role attitudes. *American Sociological Review*, 43, 541-557.

Sperber, B.M., M. Fishbein and I. Ajzen (1980), Predicting and understanding women's occupational orientations: factors underlying choice intentions. In: Ajzen and Fishbein (eds.), 113-129.

Spieß, E. (1984), Einstellungen zur Frauenrolle und paarinternen Rollenstruktur. *Problem und Entscheidung*, 26, 65-85.

Spieß, E. (1988), *Frau und Beruf - Der Wandel des Problems in Wissenschaft und Massenmedien*. Frankfurt: Campus.

Spieß, E. *et alii* (1984), Wertwandel und generatives Verhalten - Ergebnisse einer Längsschnittstudie an jungen Ehepaaren. *Zeitschrift für Bevölkerungswissenschaft*, 10, 153-168.

Spitze, G. (1988), Women's employment and family relations: a review. *Journal of Marriage and the Family*, 50, 595-618.

Standing, G. (1978), *Labour force participation and development*. Geneva: International Labour Office.

Stelcner, M. and J. Breslaw (1985), Income taxes and the labor supply of married women in Quebec. *Southern Economic Journal*, 51, 1053-1072.

Stigler, G.J. and G.S. Becker, (1977), De gustibus non est disputandum. *American Economic Review*, 67, 76-90.

Stolzenberg, R.M. and L.J. Waite (1977), Age, fertility expectations and plans for employment. *American Sociological Review*, 42, 769-782.

Strotz, R.H. (1957), The empirical implications of a utility tree. *Econometrica*, 25, 269-280.

Strotz, R.H. (1959), The utility tree: a correction and further appraisal. *Econometrica*, 27, 482-488.

Stutenbäumer-Hübner, A. (1985), Frauen im Beruf - Benachteiligungen mit System. *Mitbestimmung*, 12, 518-575.

Suls, J. and R. Miller (1977), *Social comparison processes*. Washington DC: Hemisphere.

Sweet, J.A. (1973), *Women in the labor force*. New York: Seminar Press.

Tangri, S.S. (1977), Determinants of occupational role innovation among college women. *Journal of Social Issues*, 28, 177-199.

Tazelaar, F. (1980), *Mentale incongruenties - sociale restricties - gedrag: een onderzoek naar beroepsparticipatie van gehuwde vrouwelijke academici.* PhD-dissertation, Utrecht University, Utrecht.

Tazelaar, F. (1983), Van een klassieke attitude-gedragshypothese naar een algemeen gedragstheoretisch model. In: S. Lindenberg and F.N. Stokman (eds.), *Modellen in de sociologie.* Deventer: Van Loghum Slaterus, 112-138.

Tazelaar, F. and M. Sprengers (1985), Een sociaal-structurele en een cognitief-motivationele verklaring van de reacties van werklozen op ontslag. Report, Vakgroep Theoretische Sociologie en Methodenleer, Utrecht University.

Teachman, J.D. and D.A. Heckert (1985), The declining significance of first-birth timing. *Demography*, 22, 185-198.

Tegtmeyer, H. (1976), Die soziale Schichtung der Erwerbstätigen in der BRD. *Zeitschrift für Bevölkerungswissenschaft*, 2, 34-55.

Terhune, K.W. and S. Kaufman (1973), The family size utility function. *Demography*, 10, 599-617.

Thaler, R.H. and H.M. Shefrin (1981), An economic theory of self-control. *Journal of Political Economy*, 89, 392-406.

Thomson, E. (1983), Individual and couple utility of children. *Demography*, 20, 507-518.

Thornton, A. (1978), The relationship between fertility and income, relative income, and subjective well-being. In: J. Simon (ed.), *Research in Population Economics*. Volume 1. Greenwich: JAI Press, 261-290.

Thornton, A. and J. Kim. (1980), Perceived impact of financial considerations on childbearing in the United States. In: J. Simon and J. DaVanzo (eds.), *Research in Population Economics*. Volume 2. Greenwich: JAI Press, 351-363.

Townes, B. *et alii* (1980), Family building: a social psychological study of fertility decisions. *Population and Environment*, 3, 210-220.

Turchi, B.A. (1975), *The demand for children: the economics of fertility in the United States*. Cambridge: Ballinger.

Turchi, B.A. (1979), Fertility as consumption. *Journal of Consumer Research*, 5, 293-296.

Turchi, B.A. (1981), A comprehensive micro theory of fertility. In: W. Molt, H.A. Hartmann and P. Stringer (eds.), *Advances in economic psychology*. Heidelberg: Edition Meyn, 197-210.

Turchi, B.A. (1983), *Estimating the cost of children in the United States.* Final report to the National Institute of Child Health and Human Development. Chapel Hill: Carolina Population Center.

Turchi, B.A. (1984), Rural development policy and fertility: a framework for analysis at the household level. In: W.A. Schutjer and C.S. Stokes (eds.), *Rural development and human fertility in less developed countries*. New York: MacMillan, 97-120.

Turchi, B.A. (1986), *The time cost of American children*. Final Report to the National Institute of Child Health and Human Development. Chapel Hill: Carolina Population Center.

Tversky, A. (1969), Intransitivity of preferences. *Psychological Review*, 76, 31-48.

Tversky, A. (1972), Elimination by aspects: a theory of choice. *Psychological Review*, 79, 281-299.

Udry, J.R. (1982), The effect of normative pressures on fertility. *Population and Environment*, 5, 109-122.

Ullman-Margalit, E. (1977), *The emergence of norms*, Oxford: Oxford University Press.

United Nations (1983), *Report of the meeting on population, Sofia, 6-12 October 1983*. Doc. nr. ECE/AC.9/2. Geneva: United Nations.

Van Horn, S.H. (1988), *Women, work, and family 1900-1986*. New York: New York University Press.

Van Loo, M.F. and R.P. Bagozzi (1984), Labor force participation and fertility: a social analysis of their antecedents and simultaneity. *Human Relations*, 37, 941-967.

Veenman, J. (1983), Arbeidssociologie in wording. *Beleid en Maatschappij*, 10, 202-211.

Veevers, J.E. (1973), Voluntarily childless wives. *Sociology and Social Research*, 57, 356-366.

Veron, J. (1988), Activité féminine et structure familiale: quelle dépendance ? *Population*, 43, 103-120.

Vinokur-Kaplan, D. (1977), Family planning decision-making: a comparison and analysis of parents' considerations. *Journal of Comparative Family Studies*, 8, 79-98.

Vinokur-Kaplan, D. (1978), To have or not to have another child: family planning attitudes, intentions and behavior. *Journal of Applied Social Psychology*, 8, 29-46.

van Vonderen, M. (1987), *Werken, moeder worden en carrière maken*. Maastricht: Van Gorcum.

de Vries, N.K. (1988), *Gelijkheid en complementariteit*. PhD-dissertation, Groningen University.

Waite, L.J., G.W. Haggstrom and D.E. Kanouse (1984), The effect of the first birth on the nature and extent of women's and men's employment. Paper presented at the PAA Annual Meeting 1984.

Waite, L.J. and R.M. Stolzenberg (1976), Intended childbearing and labor force participation of young women: insights from nonrecursive models. *American Sociological Review*, 41, 235-252.

Wales, T.J. and A.D. Woodland (1980), Sample selectivity and the estimation of labor supply functions. *International Economic Review*, 21, 437-468.

Warshaw, P.R., B.H. Sheppard and J. Hartwick (forthcoming), The intention and self-prediction of goals and behaviour. In: R.P. Bagozzi (ed.), *Advances in marketing communication research*. Greenwich: JAI Press.

Watson, D. and A. Tellegen (1985), Toward a consensual structure of mood. *Psychological Bulletin*, 98, 219-235.

Weber, M. (1958), Class, status, party. In: H.H. Gerth and C.W. Mills (eds.), *From Max Weber*. New York: Galaxy, 180-195.

von Weizsäcker, C.C. (1984), The influence of property rights on tastes. *Journal of Institutional and Theoretical Economics* (ZgS), 140, 90-95.

Werner, P.D., S.E. Middlestadt-Carter and T.J. Crawford (1975), Having a third child. Predicting behavioral intentions. *Journal of Marriage and the Family*, 37, 348-358.

Westoff, C.F., R.G. Potter Jr., P.C. Sagi and E.G. Michler (1961), *Family growth in metropolitan America*. Princeton: Princeton University Press.

Westoff, C.F. and N.B. Ryder (1977), The predictive validity of reproductive intentions. *Demography*, 14, 431-453.

Wilbrink-Griffioen, D., A. Elzinga and I. van Vliet (1988), Kinderopvang en arbeidsparticipatie van vrouwen. In: R.J. van Amstel, E. Slot and V.C. Vrooland (eds.), *Een kind krijgen en blijven werken*. Amsterdam: Nederlands Instituut voor Arbeidsomstandigheden, 129-146.

Willekens, F. (1988), A life course perspective on household dynamics. In: N. Keilman, A. Kuijsten and A. Vossen (eds.), *Modelling household formation and dissolution*. Oxford: Clarendon Press, 87-107.

Williams, R.M. (1975), Relative deprivation. In: L. Coser (ed.), *The idea of social structure*, New York: Harcourt Brace Jovanovich.

Willis, R.J. (1973), A new approach to the economic theory of fertility. *Journal of Political Economy*, 81, S14-S69.

Willis, R.J. (1974), A new approach to the economic theory of fertility behavior. In: T.W. Schultz (ed.), 25-75.

Willis, R.J. (1987), What have we learned from the economics of the family ? *American Economic Review Papers and Proceedings*, 77, 68-81.

Witt, U. (1987), Familienökonomie - Einige nicht-neoklassische Aspekte. In: H. Todt (ed.), *Die Familie Gegenstand sozialwissenschaftlicher Forschung*. Berlin: Duncker und Humblot, 63-84.

Wright, P.L. (1974), The harassed decision maker: time pressures, distractions, and the use of evidence. *Journal of Applied Psychology*, 59, 555-561.

Wright, P.L. and F. Barbour (1977), Phased decision strategies: sequels to an initial screening. In: M.K. Starr and M. Zeleny (eds.), *Multiple criteria decision making*. Amsterdam: North Holland, 91-109.

Yamagishi, T. (1986), The provision of a sanctioning system as a public good. *Journal of Personality and Social Psychology*, 51, 110-116.

Zellner, H. (1975), The determinants of occupational segregation. In: C. Lloyd (ed.), *Sex, discrimination, and the division of labor*. New York: Columbia University Press, 125-145.

Zerubavel, E. (1981), *Hidden rhythms: schedules and calendars in social life*. Berkeley: University of California Press.

Zimmermann, K.F. (1985), *Familienökonomie: theoretische und empirische Untersuchungen zur Frauenerwerbstätigkeit und Geburtenentwicklung*. Berlin: Springer-Verlag.

Zimmermann, K.F. (1986), Effiziente Allokation des Familienbudgets. In: K.F. Zimmermann (ed.), *Demographische Probleme der Haushaltsökonomie*. Bochum: Brockmeyer, 126-140.

Zimmermann, K.F. (1987), The variety of goods and fertility decline. Mimeo, University of Pennsylvania, Philadelphia.

Zimmermann, K.F. (1988), *Wurzeln der modernen ökonomischen Bevölkerungstheorie in der deutschen Forschung um 1900*. Jahrbücher für Nationalökonomie und Statistik, 205, 116-130.

Zimmermann, K.F. (1989a), Optimum population: an introduction. In: K.F. Zimmermann (ed.), *Economic theory of optimal population*. Heidelberg: Springer-Verlag, 1-8.

Zimmermann, K.F. (1989b), Die Konkurrenz der Genüsse: ein Brentano-Modell des Geburtenrückgangs. *Zeitschrift für Wirtschafts- und Sozialwissenschaften*, 109, 467-483.

Zimmermann, K.F. and J. De New (1990), Labor market restrictions and the role of preferences in family economics. Discussion Paper, University of Munich.

Richard P. Bagozzi (1946) is Dwight F. Benton Professor of Marketing and Behavioural Science in Management at the School of Business Administration, University of Michigan, USA. He obtained his PhD from Northwestern University in 1976. He is the author of various scientific papers published in journals like the British Journal of Social Psychology, Journal of Consumer Research and Journal of Applied Psychology.

Sabien Bauwens (1964) obtained her PhD in 1987 at the University of Ghent, Belgium. After having worked with the Population and Family Study Centre in Brussels, she is currently Research Fellow at the Faculty of Medical Psychology at the University of Ghent.

Herwig Birg (1939) is Professor of Demography and Director of the Institute for Population Research and Social Policy, University of Bielefeld, Germany; Lecturer at the Berlin Technical University; and Fellow of the German Institute for Economic Research. He obtained his PhD in 1970 from the Free University, and his Habilitation Degree in 1979 from the Technical University, both in Berlin. He is one of the pioneers of the biographic approach in demography.

Thomas K. Burch (1934) is Professor of Sociology and Director of the Population Studies Centre, University of Western Ontario, Canada. He has a PhD from Princeton University, obtained in 1962. His main research area is the behavioural foundation of demographic phenomena, particularly in family demography.

John P. De New (1965) graduated in 1988 with an MA in economics from the University of Toronto, Canada. Currently he is a research economist at the University of Mannheim, Germany, where he co-authored several conference papers with Klaus F. Zimmermann.

Freddy Deven (1947) is Senior Research Fellow at the Population and Family Study Centre in Brussels, Belgium. He obtained his PhD in 1984 from the Catholic University of Leuven with a dissertation on "Child wish and parenthood: a large-scale survey". His main research area is in the organization and analysis of fertility surveys.

John F. Ermisch (1947) obtained his PhD in economics from the University of Kansas at Lawrence, USA. Since 1986 he is Senior Research Officer at the National Institute of Economic and Social Research in London, UK. He is also Co-Director of the Human Resources Research Programme at the Centre for Economic Policy Research, London. His publications, many in the field of population economics, include articles in the European Economic Review, the Journal of Human Resources and the Journal of Population Economics.

Evert van Imhoff (1959) is Senior Research Fellow at the Netherlands Inter-disciplinary Demographic Institute. In 1988 he obtained his PhD from the Erasmus University Rotterdam with a dissertation published under the title "Optimal economic growth and non-stable population". His publications, in economics and demography, include articles in the Journal of Human Resources, the Journal of Population Economics and Mathematical Population Studies.

Jenny de Jong-Gierveld (1938) is Director of the Netherlands Interdisciplinary Demographic Institute and Professor of Social Research Methodology, Faculty of Social Sciences, Vrije Universiteit Amsterdam. She obtained her PhD in 1969 from the Vrije Universiteit Amsterdam with a dissertation on "The unmarried: the living conditions and life experiences of unmarried elderly men and women". Her publications include articles in the Journal of Personality and Social Psychology, Comprehensive Gerontology, and the Journal of Social and Personal Relationships.

Siegwart M. Lindenberg (1941) is Professor of Theoretical Sociology at Groningen University, Netherlands. In 1971 he obtained his PhD in Sociology from Harvard University with a dissertation on "Aspects of the cognitive representation of social structures".

Alice Nakamura (1945) is Professor at the Faculty of Business, University of Alberta at Edmonton, Canada. She obtained her PhD from The Johns Hopkins University in 1973. Her publications, generally written together with her husband Masao Nakamura, are in the field of labour economics and include articles in Econometrica, the Journal of Economic Behavior and Organization, and the Journal of Social Issues.

Masao Nakamura (1945) is Professor at the Faculty of Business, University of Alberta at Edmonton, Canada. He obtained his PhD from The Johns Hopkins University in 1972. His publications, many of them written together with his wife Alice Nakamura, are in the field of labour economics and also on the behaviour of Japanese and US firms.

Friedemann W. Nerdinger (1950) obtained his PhD from the University of Munich in 1989 with a dissertation titled "The world of advertisement". Since 1983 he is research assistant at the Institute of Organizational Psychology, University of Munich, Germany. Her research interests are population research, values, socialization in organizations and problems of service industries.

Lutz von Rosenstiel (1938) is Professor and Director of the Institute of Organizational Psychology, University of Munich, Germany. He obtained his PhD in 1968 and his Habilitation Degree in 1974, both from the University of Munich. He is the editor of several volumes in the field of applied psychology and also of the Zeitschrift für Arbeits- und Organisationspsychologie.

Jacques J. Siegers (1948) is Professor of Economics at Utrecht University, Netherlands, and Coordinator of the Centre for Interdisciplinary Research on Labour Market and Distribution Issues, Utrecht, Netherlands. His PhD was obtained in 1985 with a dissertation on "Labour supply and fertility: a microeconomic analysis". He is the author of various papers in the fields of demography, economics, social sciences and statistics, including articles in De Economist, the European Sociological Review and the European Journal of Population.

Erika Spieß (1954) obtained her PhD from the University of Munich in 1988 with a dissertation titled "Woman and profession". Since 1981 she is research assistant at the Institute of Organizational Psychology, University of Munich, Germany. Her research interests include population psychology, processes of personal selection and the problem of women's professional achievement.

Boone A. Turchi (1941) is Associate Professor of Economics at the University of North Carolina, Chapel Hill, USA. He obtained his PhD in economics in 1973 from the University of Michigan at Ann Arbor. His publications include articles and monographs in the fields of the economics of fertility, the estimation of the cost of children, and the impact of children on married women's labour force participation.

M. Frances Van Loo (1942) is Associate Professor of Economic Analysis and Public Policy at the The Haas School of Business, University of California at Berkeley, USA. She obtained her PhD from UC Berkeley in 1971. Her articles, many of which are the result of collaboration with Richard P. Bagozzi, include papers on the impact of preferences on economic and social behaviour.

Frans J. Willekens (1946) is Professor of Demography at Utrecht University and Groningen University, Netherlands, and Deputy Director of the Netherlands Interdisciplinary Demographic Institute. In 1976 he obtained his PhD from Northwestern University with a dissertation on "Analytics of multiregional population distribution policy". His research interests include multistate demography, stochastics processes in demography, and demographic software.

Klaus F. Zimmermann (1952) is Professor of Economics at the University of Munich, Germany. In 1984 he obtained his PhD from the University of Mannheim with a dissertation published under the title "Familienökonomie" [Family Economics], and in 1987 his Habilitation Degree, also in Mannheim. He is the author or editor of several books and various papers, including articles published in Econometrica, the American Economic Review and the Review of Economics and Statistics. He is also the managing editor of the Journal of Population Economics.

K. F. Zimmermann, University of Mannheim (Ed.)

Economic Theory of Optimal Population

With contributions by numerous experts

1989. IX, 182 pp. 19 figs. (Microeconomic Studies)
Hardcover DM 69,– ISBN 3-540-50792-2

The notion of optimum population has attracted the attention of economists ever since economics was made a science. Roots can be traced back to ancient Greece. The topic has recently found rising interest among population economists and demographers. The economic concept of optimum population seeks to define the population size, which maximizes a welfare criterion of the society. The purpose of this book is to outline this concept from a micro and macro perspective and to link it with issues of technical progress, social security, limited resources and migration. It treats fertility endogenously and studies its welfare and policy implications. The emphasis is on a rigorous theoretical treatment of the subject using the modern growth and welfare theory as well as the new classical micro model of the family.

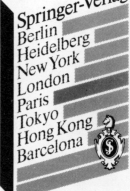

Springer-Verlag
Berlin
Heidelberg
New York
London
Paris
Tokyo
Hong Kong
Barcelona

A. Wenig, Fernuniversität Hagen;
K. F. Zimmermann, University of Mannheim
(Eds.)

Demographic Change and Economic Development

1989. XII, 325 pp. 45 figs.
(Studies in Contemporary Economics)
Softcover DM 71,- ISBN 3-540-51140-7

In recent years, population economics has become increasingly popular in both economic and policy analysis. For the inquiry into the long term development of an economy, the interaction between demographic change and economic activity cannot be neglected without omitting major aspects of the problems. This volume helps to further developments in theoretical and applied demographical economics covering the issues of demographic change and economic development.

W. Schmähl, Free University of Berlin (Ed.)

Redefining the Process of Retirement

An International Perspective

1989. XI, 179 pp. 16 figs. Hardcover DM 78,-
ISBN 3-540-50826-0

Past and future development as well as possibilities for influencing the process of retirement are discussed, in particular effects on the labour market (supply and demand, behaviour of workers and firms, concerning human resource management and occupational pensions), financing of social security and income of workers. Decisions concerning earlier or postponed, full or partial retirement are the main topic stressing the central role of firms' decisions depending e. g. on their view of the productivity of the elderly. Reports on Scandinavian countries (Sweden, Denmark, Finland) in particular on their approach for partial retirement are included as well as papers discussing possibilities to stop the trend of early exit from the labour force and how to give incentives for a longer working life (e. g. by changes in social security). These topics are discussed in the view of structural changes in demography, economy and society, using – among others – the US and West Germany as examples.

E. van Imhoff, The Hague

Optimal Economic Growth and Non-Stable Population

1989. IX, 218 pp. 27 figs.
(Studies in Contemporary Economics)
Softcover DM 53,- ISBN 3-540-51556-9

This book studies the consequences of demographic change for optimal economic growth in a closed economy. It connects the analytical tools of traditional growth theory with the actual demographic experience of most industrialized countries. A natural way of incorporating the demographic structure into growth models is by making the model one of overlapping generations, thus allowing for explicit analysis of demographic forces as potential sources of non-stationarities in economic development.
The book offers a number of economic growth models with which the effects on social welfare of demography, investment in physical and human capital, and technical progress can be analyzed. Using these models, rules for optimal economic policy can be derived. The study formulates general guidelines for long-run economic and educational policy, given the available demographic projections.
Two main conclusions are reached. First, a fall in fertility has a beneficial effect on consumption per capita, provided that the population growth rate does not pass below a certain (probably negative) critical level. Second, investment in education is a good substitute for population growth: when the population growth rate falls, investment in education becomes more attractive.

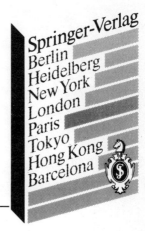

Springer-Verlag
Berlin
Heidelberg
New York
London
Paris
Tokyo
Hong Kong
Barcelona